SECRET TIPS TO ULTIMATE BEAUTY

SECRET TIPS TO ULTIMATE BEAUTY

VIJAYA KUMAR

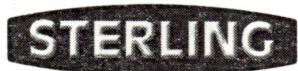

STERLING PAPERBACKS
An imprint of
Sterling Publishers (P) Ltd.
A-59, Okhla Industrial Area, Phase-II,
New Delhi-110020.
Tel: 26387070, 26386209; Fax: 91-11-26383788
E-mail: mail@sterlingpublishers.com
www.sterlingpublishers.com

Secret Tips to Ultimate Beauty
© 2006, Sterling Publishers (P) Ltd
ISBN 978 81 207 7039 3
Reprint 2007, 2008, 2009, 2010, 2012, 2014

All rights are reserved.
No part of this publication may be reproduced, stored in a retrieval system or transmitted, in any form or by any means, mechanical, photocopying, recording or otherwise, without prior written permission of the original publisher.

Printed in India
Printed and Published by Sterling Publishers Pvt. Ltd.,
New Delhi-110 020.

Contents

1. General Health — 7
2. Skin Care — 55
3. Care of Face and Neck — 66
4. Mouth, Teeth and Chin Care — 73
5. Care of Eyes — 77
6. Hair Care — 82
7. Care of Arms and Hands — 91
8. Care of Knees and Feet — 96
9. Beauty Aids — 98

Chapter One
General Health

Acidity

1. Take a glass of water with a piece of jaggery dissolved in it, after meals, and any time acidity occurs.
2. Coconut water taken thrice a day keeps away acidity.
3. Watermelon and cucumber slices taken every hour relieves one of acidity.
4. Soak a teaspoon of wheat in half a glass of water at night. Drink the water in the morning. This gives relief from acidity for a long time.
5. Make a banana shake of one banana and a glass of milk. Drinking this gives immediate relief.
6. To get relief from acidity, drink the juice of one lemon mixed in a glass of water every morning.
7. Cook four or five neem leaves with any vegetable every day for a week, and eat it to be cured of acidity.
8. Dry a piece of neem bark and powder it. Add a tablespoon of it to five cups of water and boil it until the quantity reduces to two cups. Strain the liquid, and drink thrice daily in small quantities.
9. Grind together coriander seeds, green chillies, grated coconut, ginger, and black grapes without seeds. Eat a spoon of this chutney after each meal.

Anaemia

1. Mix together two teaspoons each of honey, lemon juice and gooseberry juice. Add a cup of water and drink on an empty stomach.
2. Mix a tablespoon of gooseberry juice with a ripe, mashed banana. Consume this thrice a day.
3. Extract juice from an orange. Mix it with a mashed banana. Take this twice daily.
4. A banana taken with a tablespoon of honey does wonders to cure one of anaemia.
5. Drink a cup of apple juice on an empty stomach in the morning, and once before going to bed.
6. Beetroot juice combined with apple juice is an excellent remedy for anaemia.
7. Mash a banana and add curd and a little sugar to it. Beat well. Take once daily for a month.
8. Soak a teaspoon of fenugreek in a cup of water overnight. Drink the water and eat the seeds.
9. A teaspoon of the juice from raw turmeric, mixed with honey, should be taken every day for the treatment of this condition.

Animal Bite

Mix together one teaspoon of black cuminseed powder with half a teaspoon of honey and take twice daily.

Anorexia (Loss of Appetite)

1. Eating a mango every day builds up your appetite.
2. Mix together a tablespoon of jaggery with half a teaspoon of pepper powder. Eat it and wash it down with a glass of water.
3. Chew a cardamom thrice a day. This increases your appetite.

4. Add two teaspoons each of honey lemon juice and gooseberry juice to a cup of water. Drink this first thing in the morning.
5. Chew a bit of fresh ginger with a jaggery piece three or four times a day.
6. Mix together a teaspoon each of black cuminseeds, fennel seeds (*saunf*), dried ginger powder and carom seeds (*ajwain*). Take a teaspoon of this with water twice a day.
7. Chewing a long piece of ginger with a little salt before meals improves one's appetite.
8. Crush a one-inch piece of ginger and boil it in one and a half cups of water. Simmer for two minutes. Add milk and sugar to taste. This can be taken frequently. Cures one of aversion to food.

Asthma

1. Chew a piece of ginger every now and then in a day to relieve one of asthma.
2. Mix equal spoons of ginger juice, honey and pomegranate juice. Take a tablespoon twice daily.
3. Dry peepal tree fruits and powder them. Take a teaspoon of this powder with water daily.
4. Take figs daily to get comfort from asthma.
5. Before going to bed at night, take half a teaspoon of cinnamon powder mixed with a teaspoon of honey.
6. Turmeric powder (a spoon) boiled in a glass of milk and taken twice daily gives relief.
7. Mix together two teaspoons of honey, half a teaspoon each of onion juice and betel leaf juice and a quarter teaspoon of asafoetida (*hing*). Have it thrice a day.
8. An infusion of basil leaves (*tulsi*), cloves and salt, and taken daily gives relief.

9. Drinking lemon juice before meals and at bed time is a good cure for asthma.
10. Boil eight flakes of garlic in half a cup of milk. Have it at night.
11. A teaspoon of ginger juice mixed with a cup of fenugreek infusion and honey is an excellent medicine for asthma.
12. Add a crushed garlic in ginger tea, and take it in the morning and at night.
13. Half a cup of bittergourd juice with a little honey, taken once a day, can cure one of asthma.
14. Chew a betel leaf with five peppercorns, one clove and a pinch of camphor.
15. Inhale steam from the water in which carom seeds have been boiled.
16. Make an infusion with a handful of drumstick leaves in a cup of water. Cool and strain. Add salt, lemon juice and pepper powder. Take this once or twice a day.
17. A teaspoon of fresh mint juice, mixed with two teaspoons each of vinegar and honey, and half a cup of carrot juice relieves one of asthmatic conditions.

Backache
1. Backache can be relieved by applying ginger paste on the afflicted area, and by gently massaging the area.
2. Gently massage the back with eucalyptus oil. Then cover the area to keep it warm.

Bad Breath
1. Take caraway seed oil orally for overcoming bad breath.
2. Chew fennel seeds frequently.
3. Chew and swallow basil leaves to keep your mouth free of bad breath.

4. Use an infusion of cinnamon to rinse your mouth.
5. A few seeds of cardamom chewed for a brief while will clear your mouth of bad breath.
6. Wrap a small piece of cinnamon in a betel leaf and chew it.
7. Soak a teaspoon of fenugreek in a cup of water for an hour. Make tea, using the water and seeds. Drinking this keeps away bad breath.
8. Use dried mint leaves that are powdered as toothpowder.
9. Mix together two tablespoons of grated ginger with one and a half tablespoon of powdered jaggery. Chew this slowly till your mouth feels fresh.
10. Chew parsley leaves, which are sure to keep your breath fresh.
11. Gargle your mouth with water in which salt and soda bicarb have been added.
12. To cure bad breath boil a few fenugreek leaves in water, and gargle with this water.
13. Gargle your mouth with a mixture of lemon juice and rose water.
14. Chew on a teaspoon of aniseeds and four or five mint leaves.
15. Brush your teeth with a mixture of pepper powder and common salt.

Bedwetting

1. Rub a piece of the tender turmeric root on a sandstone. Mix the extract with honey and give it to the child before he goes to bed.
2. Let the child eat a walnut and five or six raisins before going to bed.

Bladder Stones

Boil two figs in a cup of water. Take this infusion every day for a month.

Blood-related Problems

1. To purify your blood, take a mixture of four teaspoons each of basil leaves juice and buttermilk on an empty stomach every morning.
2. Take a mixture of one tablespoon of gooseberry juice and a ripe, mashed banana twice a day for a month to combat blood deficiency.
3. Chewing a few young leaves of the peepal tree, and swallowing their juice is said to purify blood.
4. Soak three dry figs in a cup of water overnight. Take this, water and figs, with milk in the morning.

Blood Pressure, High

1. Take pepper powder mixed with a little butter on an empty stomach in the morning for nearly two months.
2. Swallow a flake of garlic with warm water on an empty stomach.
3. Patients suffering from high blood pressure can derive a lot of benefit by taking a tablespoon of neem leaf juice twice a day.
4. High blood pressure can be cured by eating the kernel of the seeds of waterwelon.
5. Take a mixture of equal quantities of ginger juice, cumin powder and honey twice a day.
6. Extract juice from a bunch of curry leaves. Mix with a lot of boiled water. Strain and drink a glass of it on an empty stomach every day for a month.

7. Eating apples every day is a sure way of bringing down the high pressure.
8. Consume plenty of coconut water and butter-milk.
9. Drink coriander juice made from fresh leaves and mixed with water thrice a day.

Blood Pressure, Low

Crush the leaves of 10-15 basil leaves. Mix with one teaspoon honey. Have this thrice a day.

Blood Sugar

Take a couple of garlic flakes every day for a month.

Body Odour

1. Mix half a teaspoon of dry ginger powder with a teaspoon of gingelly oil and a glass of milk. Consume this every day for three days.
2. Take an infusion of 10-15 basil leaves every morning for a month.
3. Mix a little sandalwood powder in a glass of water. Sprinkle this on the body. A good remedy for body odour caused by sweating.
4. The tea made from fenugreek seeds, taken regularly, gives relief from body odours.

Burns

1. Apply honey or ink to reduce the burning sensation if your hand gets burnt.
2. If you mash a banana, and apply it on the burn, it will have a cooling effect, and blisters too won't appear.
3. For burns, apply a solution of sugar and water in the absence of any other remedy within reach.

4. Soda bicarb made into a very thin paste and applied at once on the burns will bring relief.
5. Apply a little coconut oil on the burn every half an hour, and leave it open. The burn will heal soon enough.
6. If you apply egg white on the burns, blisters will not form.
7. Rub ice cubes on the affected area, then apply a solution of milk and honey to prevent blister formation.
8. Mix an egg white with equal quantity of glycerine. Soak a strip of linen in it and keep this on the affected part.
9. If you have scalded your hand, apply soap lather on it till you get relief.
10. Apply toothpaste on the burnt area. This prevents blister formation.
11. Plenty of cold water can sharply cut down the degree of burns.
12. For minor burns and scalds, cold tea provides instant relief.
13. Keep a slice of potato on the burn.
14. Fresh juice of fenugreek leaves mixed with lemon juice can be applied over burns.
15. Mix together four teaspoons each of coconut oil and lemon juice. With a spoon churn it till it becomes white. Apply on the affected part.
16. Make a paste of curry leaves and apply on the burn.
17. Rub a thin layer of honey on the burnt area and cover with a dressing. Repeat after every three hours till you get relief.
18. Immediately apply glycerine on the affected area.
19. Make an infusion with neem bark in four cups of water. Shake the bottle well. Apply the froth on the scar formed by burns every day till it fades.

20. Rub the bark of peepal tree with water on a sandstone. Mix the paste with gingelly oil and apply on the burn.
21. Extract juice from a banana stem and mix it with an equal quantity of ghee. Apply on the burn.
22. Dry tamarind leaves in a pan over fire. Powder and mix with gingelly oil and apply over the burnt area.

Bronchitis

1. Mix together three teaspoons of honey and a teaspoon of garlic oil. Taken thrice a day, a child will get relief from bronchial problem.
2. Mix together a teaspoon of asafoetida powder, two teaspoons of honey, a quarter teaspoon of onion juice and a teaspoon of betel leaf juice. This mixture is beneficial both for the prevention and treatment of bronchitis.
3. Eating fennel seeds with figs is a good medicine for bronchitis.
4. Massage the back of the chest with mustard oil mixed with a little camphor.
5. Inhalation of eucalyptus vapour helps in the treatment of bronchitis.

Cataract

Mix a teaspoon of fresh lemon juice with an equal quantity of rose water. Put this in the eyes.

Chest Congestion

1. Boil two tablespoons of fennel seeds in a cup of water till the water is reduced to half cup. Strain and take a tablespoon of it twice a day.
2. Chew a betel leaf with five peppercorns and salt.
3. Make an infusion with a teaspoon each of carom seeds powder and turmeric powder in half a litre of water. Take a tablespoon of this with a teaspoon of honey.

4. Mix a teaspoon of camphor in half a cup of warm coconut oil. Apply on the chest.
5. Mix half a teaspoon of mustard powder with a teaspoon of honey. Eat this twice daily.
6. Apply the paste of powdered nutmeg and gingelly oil on the chest for instant relief.
7. Mix equal quantities of rice flour and mustard powder in water to form a watery mustard powder. Boil till thick. Spread on a clean piece of cloth, and foment the back and front of the chest.

Cholera

1. To take preventive measures against cholera, chew 10-15 basil leaves with peppercorns daily.
2. Give the patient onion juice every hour.
3. Smear neem oil on a betel leaf and chew the leaf four times a day.
4. Boil a few cloves in water until the water is reduced by half. Take this daily.
5. Grind an onion with seven peppercorns and have it daily.

Cholesterol

1. To reduce cholesterol, blend a glass of coconut water with 200 gms papaya. Drink this every morning on an empty stomach.
2. Use sunflower oil for cooking instead of solid fats.
3. Make an infusion with two teaspoons of coriander seed powder and one cup water.
4. Blend an onion with a cup of buttermilk in a mixie. Add a quarter teaspoon of pepper powder and drink this.
5. Swallow three flakes of garlic every day. This is beneficial in reducing cholesterol substantially.

6. Make an infusion with fenugreek seeds and water. Have this daily to lower your cholesterol.

Cold

1. Take pineapple to build up resistance against colds.
2. Apply mustard oil on the bridge of the nose to relieve congestion in the nose.
3. Lemon juice in hot water with honey is a good antidote for an incipient cold.
4. Keep a cut onion in your bedroom, and you are not likely to catch a cold at night.
5. Raw onions eaten twice a day will help to clear stuffed nostrils.
6. To check an imminent sneeze, press a finger on the middle of the upper lip. The sneeze will subside.
7. Consume daily a paste made of honey, ghee, turmeric powder and salt till the cold has gone.
8. Take a few leaves of basil with honey.
9. Take the mixture made of gooseberry powder, ginger powder and water twice daily.
10. To treat a recurring cold, chew four black peppercorns on an empty stomach in the mornings.
11. For a child with severe cold, mix a pinch of common salt with a teaspoon of lukewarm mustard oil, and apply on his chest morning and night.
12. Inhaling the fumes from a turmeric stick heated over the fire is an excellent remedy for cold.
13. For acute cold, boil a pinch of turmeric and a teaspoon of pepper powder in milk. Have at bed time for three days.
14. Make an infusion with ginger and water. Sweeten with sugar and drink it hot.

15. Make an infusion with cuminseeds and ginger powder in water. Drink twice a day.
16. Boil a flake of garlic, a small piece of ginger, five peppercorns (crushed) and ten basil leaves in a cup of water for two minutes. Strain. Add a teaspoon of honey and have it every morning.
17. Extract the juice from four basil leaves and a betel leaf. Mix it with honey and take it daily till the cold disappears.
18. Grate a piece of ginger. Put the gratings in a glass. Squeeze half a lemon into it and top it up with hot water and a little honey. Stir well and drink the contents.
19. Prepare an infusion with ginger paste, cloves and cinnamon. Add honey and drink it. Make a paste of nutmeg, poppy seeds and milk, and apply on the forehead and nose for quick relief from a running nose.
20. Boil tamarind water with a little salt and half a teaspoon of ghee. Drink this to clear nasal blockage.

Corns

1. Place a cut lemon piece on the corn and bandage the area. Leave it overnight.
2. Massage castor oil well on the corns twice a day for a month.
3. Make a poultice of cloves and garlic, both crushed and tied over the corns. Keep it overnight.

Constipation

1. Soak three basil leaves in a glass of water overnight, and drink it the first thing in the morning.
2. Eat a ripe banana before going to bed.
3. Take a thick slice of papaya before retiring for the night.
4. Drink hot water with lemon juice early in the morning.

5. Rub a little salt, cumin powder and pepper powder on a sliced papaya piece and eat it twice daily.
6. To cure one of chronic constipation, drink the juice of bottlegourd mixed with a little salt.
7. Drink soup every night to be cured of constipation.
8. Drink at least four glasses of water on waking up in the morning.
9. Soak eight dates overnight. Run them in a blender with water, and drink on an empty stomach.
10. Soak 15 raisins overnight. Drink the water and chew the raisins first.
11. When in season, eat mangoes.
12. The seeds of basil plants are laxative, and should be taken internally.
13. Chewing cuminseeds after meals prevents constipation.
14. Make an infusion of tamarind, black pepper, cloves, and cardamoms with water. Drinking this relieves one of constipation.

Cough

1. A simple home remedy for cough is to have honey in a hot drink before bed time.
2. Turmeric powder boiled in milk and taken internally relieves cough.
3. Dry cough can be cured by gradually swallowing a mixture of cuminseed powder mixed with ghee.
4. All kinds of cough can be cured by drinking the juice of ashgourd mixed with a little hot water.
5. To relieve fits of coughing due to dryness in the throat, suck a few peppercorns.
6. Use an infusion of ginger thrice a day.

7. Put a grain of salt into your mouth to stop a persistent cough.
8. Taking a mixture of lemon juice honey and glycerine is an effective remedy for cough.
9. Suck a whole clove without chewing it to soothe a cough.
10. Chew a few leaves of basil, a betel leaf and a clove together.
11. Boil a handful of tamarind leaves in water with half a teaspoon of asafoetida and a teaspoon of salt. Drink this thrice daily.
12. Cut a ripe banana into four pieces. Fry in ghee till brown. Cool and eat twice daily.
13. Have an infusion of basil leaves every morning.
14. Make an infusion with fenugreek leaves, ginger and honey. Drink it thrice daily.
15. Boil an onion, five basil leaves, five peppercorns and two cloves in one and a half cups of water till it is reduced to one cup. Drink it hot thrice a day.
16. Three peppercorns with a pinch of salt and black cumin can be taken for relief.
17. Mix together four teaspoons of jaggery and a teaspoon of pepper powder. Make into small balls and suck four of these each day.
18. Apples bring great relief to a person with dry cough.
19. Mix a tablespoon of poppy seeds with a teaspoon of honey and ten tablespoons of coconut milk. Take every night before going to bed.
20. An infusion made with the bark of neem is said to cure cough.

Cramps
1. Apply olive oil on the affected parts.
2. Apply clove oil as poultice on the affected area.

Cuts and Bruises
1. Soak a cotton wad in iodine, and dab lightly on the injured area.
2. A small piece of alum stops the flow of blood from a cut.
3. Apply the juice of basil leaves to stem the flow of blood from a cut.
4. Crush a betel leaf with lemon juice, and apply on the cut.
5. Application of coffee powder on a profusely bleeding cut stops the blood flow at once.
6. Press a little turmeric powder, an antiseptic, on the cut.
7. If a glass piece or wooden splinter gets embedded in your skin or cut, apply a layer of fevicol. When it dries and becomes transparent, peel off the layer carefully. The embedded piece will come out whole.
8. Dab the milky sap from the leaf of the peepal tree on a cut to cure it soon.
9. Put sugar on your bleeding finger or lip to stop the bleeding.
10. A cotton swab dipped in brandy acts as an antiseptic.
11. All kinds of cuts can be quickly cured by the application of honey.
12. Place a sliced onion on the bruise, but not on broken skin.
13. Grind peepal leaves with a little jaggery and apply on bruises to reduce pain.
14. Saffron can be used as a dressing for bruises.

Dehydration

1. Mix together a quarter teaspoon of salt, two teaspoons lemon juice and three teaspoons sugar in a cup of water, and drink this.
2. Make an infusion of half a nutmeg in two cups of water. Mix a teaspoon of this infusion in a cup of fresh coconut water. Drink this thrice a day.
3. Mix a teaspoon of lemon juice in a glass of coconut water. Drink this thrice a day.

Delivery Problems

1. Taking lemon juice with a little sugar daily from the fourth month of pregnancy will ensure easy delivery.
2. Mix together a quarter teaspoon of pepper powder, one teaspoon of honey and three teaspoons of lemon juice in one cup of water. Drink for three months.
3. Eating bananas daily will ensure an easy delivery.
4. A decoction made of cinnamon has been found valuable in reducing labour pain during child-birth.

Dental Problems

1. Use commercial clove oil for toothache.
2. In case of toothache, suck one or two cloves.
3. Brushing teeth with a piece of apple will keep toothaches at bay.
4. Burn a turmeric stick and powder it. Use this powder with salt for cleaning the teeth for healthy teeth and gums.
5. A pinch of salt applied to the aching tooth will bring temporary relief.
6. Raw onions eaten daily is good for maintaining strong and healthy teeth.

7. Lemon or orange rind powder makes an ideal tooth powder.
8. If your teeth have turned sour, try chewing tender mango leaves.
9. Lemon juice makes an excellent teeth cleaner.
10. Dabbing vanilla essence on the aching tooth gives immediate relief.
11. Mix a little asafoetida powder with a little salt and a small piece of raw ginger. Keep it on the crevice where the ache occurs.
12. Grind basil leaves with a little pepper. Apply this on the affected tooth or cavity.
13. Pyorrhoea (inflammation of the gums) can be cured by eating oranges daily, and rubbing the gums with the peels.
14. Mix alum with a little honey to a paste and rub on the weak or bleeding gums.
15. Apply a little sandalwood oil on the affected tooth to get relief from pain.
16. Make an infusion with neem leaves and use it for rinsing your mouth. Gives instant relief from toothache.
17. Apply clove oil mixed with pepper powder on the affected part.
18. Apply nutmeg oil on the affected tooth.
19. Use powdered shells of almonds as toothpowder.
20. Boil eight betel leaves in a litre of water. Wash the mouth frequently with this water to cure swelling and pain in the gums.
21. Chewing coconut pieces with a little jaggery strengthens gums and prevents tooth decay.
22. Rub burnt ginger mixed with salt over the teeth to cure dental sensitiveness caused by eating sour fruits.
23. The fresh leaves of mint, chewed daily, is an effective antiseptic dentifrice.

Diabetes

1. Frequently drinking bittergourd juice is good for diabetics.
2. Drink half a glass of curd with a teaspoon of fenugreek powder on an empty stomach to control diabetes.
3. A tablespoon of the juice of fresh fenugreek leaves taken early in the morning controls diabetes.
4. Dates are good for controlling diabetes.
5. Take two tablespoons of water in which neem leaves have been boiled.
6. Dry and powder mango leaves. Take half a teaspoon of this powder twice a day in the morning.
7. Eating ten curry leaves every morning for three months is said to ward off diabetes that may set in due to hereditary factors.
8. Chew ten basil leaves in the morning.
9. Take half a teaspoon of turmeric powder with honey daily.
10. Take half a teaspoon of cinnamon powder with every meal to control blood sugar.

Diarrhoea

1. A teaspoon of fenugreek powder mixed with buttermilk is an effective antidote for diarrhoea.
2. Chew guava leaf for acute diarrhoea.
3. Mix a little salt with lime juice and drink it without adding water.
4. Mix a pinch of salt with a tablespoon of ginger juice, and drink it.
5. Swallow a teaspoon of fenugreek seeds with a tablespoon of curd for immediate relief from diarrhoea.
6. Mix together a teaspoon each of cuminseed powder into a thick paste. Take a teaspoon thrice a day.

7. Black tea is very effective against diarrhoea.
8. Mash a ripe banana with a pinch of salt and a teaspoon of tamarind pulp. Take this twice a day.
9. Make an infusion with a teaspoon of cuminseeds. Add a pinch of salt and a teaspoon of fresh coriander juice. Drink twice daily for three days.
10. Take milk in which three flakes of garlic have been boiled.
11. Make a paste of one green chilli with half a teaspoon of camphor and two tablespoons of lemon juice. Take a quarter teaspoon of this paste.
12. Drink a weak tea with a quarter teaspoon of cardamom powder in it.
13. Extract juice from tender curry leaves. Mix it with a teaspoon of honey and drink it.
14. Soak three teaspoons of coriander seeds overnight in water. Mix this with a cup of buttermilk and drink it.
15. Shred apple and leave for 20 minutes till brown. Eat these shreds.
16. Infuse a quarter teaspoon of nutmeg powder into a ripe banana, and eat this.
17. Grind a handful of mango flowers, mix with water, and drink.
18. Chop two apples, and boil the pieces in milk, and drink the milk with the pieces.
19. Mix together ginger powder, a pinch of salt, and jaggery. Add it to water, and drink.

Dysentery

1. Grind the tender twigs of curry leaves, and mix it in half a glass of buttermilk. Drink this four times a day.
2. Strong tea without milk or sugar is beneficial.

3. Drink buttermilk mixed with ginger powder after meals.
4. Neem leaf juice mixed with sugar is a very effective remedy for dysentery.
5. Mix ginger juice with brown sugar and take thrice a day.
6. Take a teaspoon of cuminseed powder mixed with water thrice a day.
7. Saute a teaspoon of poppy seeds to golden brown. Add with honey and take it twice a day.

Ears

1. Put a few drops of basil leaf juice in the ear to ease the pain.
2. Wash the ear with a solution of alum in water in case of pus formation.
3. Warm a quarter teaspoon of mustard oil, and pour it in the ear in which there is pain. Plug the ear with a piece of cotton.
4. Heat a little onion juice and put a few drops of it in the ear to get relief from pain.
5. Heat a little gingelly oil with a flake of garlic. Put a few drops into the ear for relief from pain.
6. Mix a few drops of honey with water, and put a few drops of it into the painful ear.
7. Put two drops of lukewarm neem oil inside the ear to clear it.
8. Extract juice from mango leaves and warm it. Put a few drops of it into the ear to clear it of infection.
9. To two teaspoons of hot mustard oil, add half a teaspoon of carom seeds and a flake of garlic. Boil till the concoction turns red. Filter and use as ear drops.
10. Warm a mixture of basil leaf juice, lemon juice and gingelly oil. Use as ear drops.

11. Apply a few drops of sandal oil in the ears to stop discharge from the ear.
12. A clove sauted in a teaspoon of gingelly oil, and three to five drops of this oil put into the ear can cure earache.
13. A few drops of ginger juice will give relief.

Eczema
1. Grind potatoes to a fine paste. Add a little lemon juice to it. Apply on the affected parts.
2. Rub a nutmeg with water against a sandstone. Apply this paste on the affected area.
3. Mix together turmeric powder, neem juice and gingelly oil, and apply on the affected areas.
4. Apply the mixture of camphor and sandal paste on the affected areas.
5. Mix a tablespoon of neem leaf powder with eight drops of neem oil. Apply on the eczema.

Epilepsy
Apply fresh lemon juice on the head and massage well before showering off.

Excess Salivation
Chewing basil leaves cures one of excess salivation provided you do it every day for two months.

Eyes
1. To get relief from eye irritation wash it with water to which is added a few drops of rose water.
2. Apply a little refined castor oil on the eyelids to be free of boils in or around the eyes.
3. Splashing cold water several times into the eyes will keep your eyes clear and perfect.

4. To lubricate dry eyes, soak cotton pads in water, squeeze out extra water, and cover the eyes with them for 20 minutes.
5. A weak solution of water and pure sugar will cleanse your eyes and improve your eyesight.
6. The juice of fenugreek leaves is an effective cure for conjunctivitis.
7. Take a ripe banana along with a little curd and water twice a day.
8. Mix together a teaspoon of tomato juice, half a teaspoon of lemon juice, a pinch of turmeric powder and a little gram flour into a paste. Apply on the dark circles around the eyes, leave it on for 10 minutes, then wash off.
9. Soak cotton pads in cucumber juice and keep on eyes for 10-15 minutes.
10. Dip two cotton pads in a solution of water and a drop of lavender oil. Squeeze out extra water, and keep them over the eyes for 10-15 minutes.
11. To improve eyesight, eat cardamom with a teaspoon of honey every day.
12. Mix basil juice with pure honey. Apply on eyes to cure related problems.
13. For night blindness eat two slices of papaya regularly.
14. An infusion of coriander seeds, used as an eye wash, relieves burning, reduces pain and swelling in conditions of conjunctivitis.
15. Bathe the sore or inflamed eye with fennel tea.

Fainting
1. If a person faints, hold a crushed onion near his nostrils.
2. To revive a person who has fainted apply a pinch of ginger powder on the nostrils.

3. A hot poultice of carom seeds may be used as dry fomentation for hands and feet.

Fatigue
1. Drink a weak tea with a quarter teaspoon of cardamom powder in it.
2. Drink a glass of lemon juice mixed with grape juice.

Fever
1. Boil orange peels in water until it is reduced to a quarter of its quantity, and drink it hot.
2. Salt a few pieces of raw papaya, and have a slice each day.
3. Drink a hot infusion of ginger powder and coriander powder.
4. An infusion of neem juice with pepper powder lowers temperature.
5. Drink tea in which a teaspoon of fenugreek seeds and honey have been added while boiling.
6. Apply sandal paste on the forehead to bring the temperature down.
7. Make an infusion of two tablespoons of fennel seeds in a cup of water, reducing the water to half its quantity while boiling. Take a tablespoon every morning.
8. In two cups of water boil eight basil leaves with a teaspoon of cardamom powder. Drink it with milk and sugar thrice a day.
9. For a feeling of feverishness, drink a cup of tender coconut water with fresh lemon juice.
10. Crush 15 basil leaves and eat this with a marble-sized piece of jaggery.
11. Grate ginger and add it to a glass of hot water with a tablespoon of lemon juice and a little honey. Drink this.

12. Crush a bark piece of neem and make an infusion with it. Drink this thrice a day.
13. Chew basil leaves with a ginger piece and a little pepper powder.
14. Boil a glass of milk with crushed garlic and take it warm when the quantity reduces by half.
15. Make an infusion of tamarind pulp in half a litre of milk with dates, sugar and cloves. Drink a cup of this.

Feet
1. Bathe tired feet in a basin of fairly hot water in which a handful of salt has been added.
2. Rub glycerine on tired feet at bedtime.
3. For relaxing tired and aching toes, try picking up marbles from the floor with your toes gripping them.
4. Add soda bicarb in hot water, and soak tired feet in them.
5. Dip your feet alternately in hot and cold waters, then massage feet with oil.
6. To be rid of foot rot between toes apply a little turmeric powder at bedtime.
7. For cracks on feet, apply a thick paste of turmeric and castor oil half an hour before bath.
8. Mix molten wax with coconut oil and apply this on cracked heels.
9. Apply sandalwood paste mixed with ghee on the cracks of heels.
10. Take internally equal quantities of carom seeds with sugar to keep the feet soft.
11. Make a paste with ghee and pepper, and eat it.
12. Take onion juice mixed with honey for a month for soft and smooth feet.

13. Rub feet with Vaseline for a smooth skin.
14. For burning sensation in feet, mash a ripe banana with curd, and take it twice a day.
15. Make a paste with bittergourd leaves and apply it on feet.
16. Apply a paste made of a handful of henna leaves and two tablespoons of lemon juice.
17. Grate bottlegourd and apply on feet, keeping it on for 20 minutes before washing off.
18. Apply a paste of ground neem leaves and turmeric on soles with cracks.
19. Massage feet with castor oil every night.
20. Apply every night a mixture of glycerine and lemon juice.
21. Make a paste of raw ginger and tender neem leaves. Apply on feet if there is fungal infection.
22. Massage swollen feet with neem oil mixed with warm milk.

Flatulence and Belching

1. Roast and grind aniseed. Mix with carom seeds and sugar. Take a spoon of it after meals.
2. Mix a teaspoon of carom seeds in a teaspoon of lemon juice. Mix this water and drink.
3. Drink a cup of hot water with half a teaspoon of ginger powder, honey and a little ghee.
4. A tea prepared with aniseed, caraway seeds and fennel seeds is beneficial in the treatment of flatulence.
5. Adding asafoetida to foodstuffs prevents flatulence.
6. One or two drops of cinnamon oil taken with half a teaspoon of sugar thrice daily acts as an antidote for flatulence.
7. An infusion with coriander seeds taken with honey is beneficial in the treatment of flatulence.

8. Drink an infusion of cuminseeds mixed with fresh coriander leaves juice and a pinch of salt.
9. Make an infusion with fennel seeds in a cup of water and drink this to treat flatulence.
10. Chewing a piece of ginger after meals regularly is an insurance against flatulence.
11. Mix mint juice with lemon juice, honey and water, and drink it thrice daily.
12. Make an infusion of tamarind pulp in water. Add pepper powder, clove and cardamom powder and a little camphor, and drink.
13. A pinch of turmeric in buttermilk is useful as an antiseptic against digestive disorders, especially flatulence.

Flu (Influenza)

1. A mixture of basil juice, ginger and honey is a good remedy for flu.
2. A tea in which fenugreek seeds have also been boiled reduces the flu condition.
3. A teaspoon of fresh ginger juice mixed with a cup of fenugreek decoction and honey to taste is an excellent mixture to reduce fever in flu.
4. For treating flu, equal amounts of onion juice and honey should be mixed, and three teaspoons of it taken daily.

Gastritis

1. Combine four peppercorns with one teaspoon of ginger powder, half a teaspoon of carom seeds and the seeds of two cardamoms. Powder these, and take a pinch with water whenever needed.
2. Regular use of garlic is very effective.
3. Take five pieces of ginger with salt during meals.

4. Powder five black peppers and five cloves. Add a cup of hot water and a pinch of salt. Drink this when the condition is acute.
5. Take a teaspoon of thyme with a quarter teaspoon of black salt in a glass of water.
6. Add a pinch of asafoetida and black salt with a quarter teaspoon of ginger powder in half a cup of warm water, and drink it.
7. A teaspoon of brandy mixed with warm water gives immediate relief from gas.
8. Make an infusion with a teaspoon of caraway seeds in a litre of water, boiled for 15 minutes on low heat. Drink a cup of this after meals.
9. A mixture of tamarind and jaggery is beneficial.

Giddiness

1. Soak cumin seeds in lemon juice overnight. Keep it in the sun till dry. Store it and use half a teaspoon in a glass of water when you feel giddy.
2. Soak a teaspoon each of coriander seeds, gooseberry powder and sandal powder in a cup of water overnight. Strain and drink the next day. This can be followed for a few days at a stretch to be free of giddiness caused by high or low blood pressure.

Headaches

1. Place a few icecubes in a polythene bag, and apply this on the forehead and temples.
2. Apply a paste of ginger powder on the forehead for quick relief.
3. Make a paste of cinnamon, peppercorns, a tiny piece of ginger and a little ginger powder. Apply on the forehead.

4. Make a paste of gooseberry pulp, and apply on the forehead and temples.
5. Grind three cloves to a fine paste. Add half a teaspoon of ginger powder, and apply on nose, forehead, etc.
6. Sniffing a muslin bag filled with roasted carom seeds relieves one of a headache.
7. For constant headaches and migraines, eat an apple with a little salt every morning.
8. Grind an onion and apply as paste on the forehead.
9. Make a paste of basil leaves, cloves and ginger powder, and apply on the forehead.
10. Mix together camphor, nutmeg powder, cardamom powder and clove powder. Take half a teaspoon of it with warm water.
11. Make a paste with basil leaves and cardamom, and apply on the forehead.
12. Mix a little camphor with sandal paste and apply on the forehead.
13. Heat a betel leaf over a candle flame and place it on the forehead.

Heart Ailments
1. Eating a lot of soya beans is very good for heart patients.
2. Carrots taken daily will prove beneficial to those having problems with the heart.
3. Mix together pomegranate seed powder, cinnamon powder and cardamom powder. Add a teaspoon of this in a glass of water, and drink.
4. Buttermilk taken instead of milk is good for heart patients.
5. For chest pain, mix two teaspoons of almond oil with one teaspoon of rose oil. Apply on the chest, and massage lightly.

6. Make an infusion with fenugreek seeds. Take it with honey twice daily.
7. Swallow a garlic flake on an empty stomach every morning.
8. An apple a day with honey will keep heart problems away.

Heart Burns
1. Drink a solution of water and jaggery.
2. Brew fennel seeds with mint leaves for 15 minutes. Drink hot.
3. Two tablespoons of honey mixed with cinnamon powder relieves one of heart burns.
4. Drink buttermilk to which a pinch of nutmeg powder and cinnamon powder have been added.
5. Drink a cup of water with a teaspoon of mint juice thrice daily.
6. Add half a teaspoon of cardamom powder to a glass of water, and drink it.

Heat Stroke
1. To get relief from heat stroke, boil raw mango, and when cool, rub the pulp on the soles of the feet.
2. Pressure cook raw mango slices. Cool and extract the soft pulp and grind to a paste. Mix with water and sugar, and drink it.

Hepatitis
Mix two teaspoons of coriander leaves juice in a cup of butter milk and take it thrice.

Hiccups
1. Hold your breath as long as you can.
2. Very slowly sip one or more glasses of water.
3. Gargle with plain water for at least a minute.

4. Pull out your tongue.
5. Swallow a spoon of sugar.
6. Swallow half a teaspoon of mustard seeds mixed with half a teaspoon of pure ghee.
7. Boil a teaspoon of cardamom powder in half a litre of water till only one cup remains. Cool, and drink when warm.
8. Suck small pieces of ginger.

Hoarseness
1. Take a teaspoon each of honey and onion juice.
2. Mix a tablespoon of honey with the seeds of a cardamom. Eat this every day.
3. Make an infusion of a teaspoon of cinnamon powder and cardamom powder in a glass of boiling water. Gargle with this water.
4. Boil two teaspoons of fennel seeds in barley water. Take it thrice a day.
5. Gargle with mint-salt decoction.

Impotence
1. Take basil leaves daily.
2. Take half a teaspoon of coriander powder with honey.
3. Swallow three flakes of garlic daily with a glass of water.

Indigestion
1. Drink hot water with ginger juice and honey.
2. Eat a little carom seeds frequently.
3. Eat a burnt garlic.
4. Mix pepper powder, lemon juice and salt, and rub on raw radish slice. Eating such slices will relieve you of indigestion.

5. Eating a ripe banana smeared with cardamom before going to bed relieves one of indigestion.
6. Drink a glass of water mixed with a teaspoon of lemon juice and a pinch of salt.
7. Eat cardamom seeds with a little sugar.
8. Heat a glass of buttermilk to which is added a little cuminseed, curry leaf and ginger powder. Drink it warm before going to bed.
9. Make an infusion of cinnamon, pepper powder and honey. A tablespoon of this after meals relieves one of indigestion.
10. Soak a teaspoon of celery seeds in buttermilk for six hours. Run this in a blender, and then drink it.
11. Take basil leaves mixed with honey twice a day, preferably first on an empty stomach.
12. Orange juice is beneficial to combat indigestion.
13. Grind cardamom seeds with ginger, cloves and coriander seeds. This is an effective remedy for indigestion.
14. A drop of clove oil added to a teaspoon of sugar and a pinch of soda bicarb is beneficial.
15. The juice of fresh coriander leaves is beneficial.

Insect Bites
1. Drink water mixed with a teaspoon of basil leaves, and also apply externally on the bitten area.
2. Apply sandal paste on the affected area.
3. Drink a cup of water that has two teaspoons of coriander juice in it.
4. Apply lemon juice diluted with water over the area.
5. The juice of the berries from curry leaves tree mixed with lemon juice is an effective fluid for external application in insect bites and stings.

Insomnia

1. A biscuit and a glass of hot milk at bed time helps many sleepless persons.
2. A raw onion eaten daily induces sound sleep.
3. Hot milk with nutmeg and honey at bedtime induces sleep.
4. A touch of perfume mixed with cologne at your nostrils at bedtime will help you sleep better.
5. Lie on your back and do deep breathing for about 15 times, and then on the side. You will easily go to sleep.
6. Take plenty of curd throughout the day.
7. Massage your head with curd before washing your hair. This ensures good sleep at night.
8. A teaspoon of fried cuminseed powder mixed with the pulp of a ripe banana can be taken at night regularly.
9. A teaspoon of honey combined with two teaspoons of fenugreek leaves juice may be taken daily.
10. Soak a tablespoon of mint leaves in a cup of water for an hour. Drink every night.
11. Soak and grind poppy seeds. Mix with coconut milk and honey, and have it every night.
12. Grind neem leaves with milk and apply over the soles. After 10 minutes wash it off.
13. Nutmeg powder mixed with gooseberry juice is an effective medicine for insomnia.

Intestinal Worms

1. Swallow a small piece of asafoetida rolled in fresh butter. This is effective in deworming.
2. Eat papayas frequently.
3. Mix a teaspoon of turmeric powder with a pinch of salt and have it first thing in the morning.

4. Fry a teaspoon of neem flowers in a teaspoon of ghee. Mix with a cup of boiled rice, and eat this twice a day.
5. Mix a teaspoon of fried fenugreek powder in water and drink thrice a day for three days.
6. Drink a glass of buttermilk to which is added a tablespoon of bittergourd juice.
7. A teaspoon of dried and powdered neem leaves mixed with jaggery should be taken every day for two weeks.
8. Prepare a hot infusion of neem bark. Take six teaspoons twice a day for a week.
9. Eat a paste of neem leaves on an empty stomach and chase it down with a glass of warm water.
10. Take pineapple juice every day.
11. An infusion made of water and cuminseeds, and taken regularly serves as a great antiseptic against hookworm infection.
12. Garlic is an excellent worm expeller.
13. Mint juice is beneficial in the treatment of threadworms, and should be taken with lemon juice and honey thrice daily.
14. About 20 drops of the juice of raw turmeric rhizomes with a pinch of salt should be taken first thing in the morning.

Itches

1. Turmeric powder mixed with powdered carom seeds and onion juice should be applied to the itches.
2. Apply a solution of ground poppy seeds, water and lemon juice on the affected areas.
3. Add two handfuls of neem leaves to a bucket of hot water and use it for your bath.

4. Mix dried and powdered neem leaves with gingelly oil. Apply on the affected areas.
5. Ground poppy seeds mixed with lemon juice should be rubbed on the affected areas.

Jaundice

1. A teaspoon of tamarind pulp with jaggery and a paste of cuminseeds should be taken thrice daily.
2. Soak peepal tree bark powder in water overnight. Drink this on an empty stomach for a few days.
3. Drink fresh buttermilk mixed with sugar candy five or six times a day.
4. Drink lemon juice frequently.
5. Mash a ripe banana and take it with a tablespoon of honey twice a day.
6. Take the infusion of a handful of lemon leaves in a cup of hot water.
7. Mix together a teaspoon each of lemon and mint juice, a tablespoon of honey and half a teaspoon of ginger juice. Take this often.
8. Mix a quarter teaspoon of turmeric in a glass of hot water, and drink this thrice daily.
9. Take four teaspoons of basil juice for two weeks.

Joint Pains (Arthritis, Rheumatism, Gout)

1. Lemon juice mixed with coconut oil soothes aching joints.
2. Two tablespoons of mustard powder dissolved in bath water does wonders for rheumatic pains.
3. Frequently eat fruits like oranges, sweet limes, grapes, apples, etc.
4. Make a paste of ginger powder with water, and heat it till warm. Apply on the rheumatic swellings of joints.

5. Take a diet of only bananas for three days. You can take up to eight or nine bananas in a day.
6. Swallow a garlic clove first thing in the morning.
7. Mix together two teaspoons of jaggery with a teaspoon of gooseberry powder, and have it twice a day.
8. Regularly massage the joints with neem oil.
9. Have four walnuts on an empty stomach for a few days.
10. Apply gingelly oil to which has been added three tablespoons of nutmeg powder.
11. Mix ginger juice with asafoetida powder and apply on the joints, and massage lightly.
12. Grind a handful of basil leaves with six peppercorns. Add a tablespoon of ghee. Take this twice a day for 20 days.
13. Try a handful of chopped ginger in 100 ml of coconut oil. Use this for massage of the joints.
14. Five drops of clove oil and 30 ml of olive oil can be applied as a liniment.
15. Crush the leaves of tamarind tree in water and make a poultice. Apply over inflamed joints.
16. Mix asafoetida with coconut oil and apply as an analgesic balm in rheumatoid arthritis.

Kidney Problems
1. Take plenty of almonds every day.
2. Make an infusion with two teaspoons of coriander powder in a glass of hot water. Add sugar and milk, and drink twice a day.
3. Eat cardamom seeds with the seeds of cucumber to obtain relief from kidney stones.

Lactation
1. A pinch of asafoetida with a teaspoon of an infusion of cloves taken thrice a day increases secretion of breast milk.
2. Take a pinch of cinnamon powder with honey.
3. Take a gruel comprising roasted fenugreek seeds, milk and sugar.
4. Eat cooked unripe papaya often.
5. Boil two teaspoons of fennel seeds in barley water and take it twice daily.
6. Add a teaspoon each of cumin powder and sugar to a cup of warm milk, and take it after dinner.
7. Eat betel leaves with aniseeds every day.

Leprosy
1. Drink milk mixed with two tablespoons of neem leaf juice for six months.
2. Take poppy seeds mixed with water thrice daily for a period of six months.

Leucoderma
Boil crushed turmeric pieces till water reduces by half. Mix with gingelly oil and boil again till only oil remains. Apply on white patches every morning and evening.

Liver Complaints
1. Tomatoes taken daily are an effective cure for liver problems.
2. Drink lemon juice with sugar daily as it is very efficacious on an upset liver.
3. Mix honey and bittergourd juice and drink it regularly.
4. Finely chop pineapple and mix with honey. Leave for four days, then eat a few pieces every day.
5. Drink pineapple juice every day.

6. Cook fenugreek leaves and eat them as they are, chased down with water.
7. Chew black basil leaves frequently.
8. Soak saffron in water and drink this often.

Malaria

Mix neem bark powder with hot water, and drink thrice a day.

Menstrual Problems

1. Add a little salt, ginger powder, a crushed garlic to a glass of water, and drink on an empty stomach to be free of the discomforting pains.
2. For painful menstruation, drink half a cup of bittergourd juice with honey.
3. Add salt to your bath water.
4. Fried and powdered asafoetida taken with a little melted sugar or jaggery gives you relief from pains.
5. Crush a hibiscus flower to a pulp and mix it in a cup of milk. Drink this to control excessive bleeding.
6. Grind together a flake of garlic, a few neem leaves and a small piece of turmeric stick. Mix it in water and drink daily to control excessive bleeding.
7. Mix together honey and sugar and take it for five days, if you have heavy bleeding.
8. To control white discharge, take honey with gooseberry juice.
9. Drink milk mixed with a teaspoon of fenugreek powder and sugar to control white discharge.
10. Boil saffron in one cup water till the water reduces by half. Drink this thrice for pains.
11. Crush the raw fruits of the peepal tree in buttermilk, and drink this twice a day to cure you of white discharge.

12. Excess bleeding can be controlled by eating a handful of roasted raw mango peel.
13. Take banana pulp mixed with sugar and honey to stop white discharge.
14. Crush a ginger piece, add honey and warm water. Drink at bed time for relief from pain.
15. Boil coriander seeds in a cup of water till the water is reduced by half. Add sugar candy and drink it warm for relief from excessive bleeding.
16. Fennel seeds regulates menstruation.
17. A tea made with mint leaves alleviates pain.

Morning Sickness

1. A cup of tea with some biscuits on waking up helps in preventing morning sickness.
2. Sip little by little ginger juice mixed with honey before you get out of bed.
3. Chewing a piece of tamarind with salt on waking up helps.
4. Half a teaspoon of cuminseed powder mixed with a teaspoon of honey before breakfast helps one fight nausea.
5. Take a teaspoon each of fresh mint juice, lemon juice, and a tablespoon of honey thrice daily.
6. Take the juice of 20 tender curry leaves with two teaspoons of lemon juice and one teaspoon of sugar in the morning.
7. Mix a pinch of nutmeg powder with a tablespoon of gooseberry juice, and take it thrice a day.

Mouth Ulcers

1. Gargle with a mixture of glycerine and rose water mixed in water.
2. Apply glycerine on the ulcer.
3. Gargle with a solution of water and alum.

4. Keep a mixture of coriander powder and honey in the mouth, and swallow it very gradually.
5. Chew basil leaves frequently.
6. For a burnt tongue, suck a spoon of sugar.
7. Gargle with a solution of potassium permanganate.
8. Massage the gums with a mixture of coconut milk and honey.
9. Mix sandal paste and lemon juice in water and use it for gargling.
10. Take tomato juice mixed with buttermilk.
11. Mix a teaspoon of neem juice with buttermilk and drink it.

Nasal Problems

1. Place a piece of newspaper over the nose to stop bleeding from the nose.
2. Eat a mixture of a little alum with sugar candy thrice a day to stop frequent nose bleeding.
3. For a stuffy nose, eat raw onions twice a day.
4. Inhale the fumes of a burnt turmeric to open clogged nostrils.
5. Add two cloves, one cardamom, half a teaspoon of ginger powder and two basil leaves to the water while making tea. Drinking this often cures a running nose.
6. Drop lemon juice in nostrils to stop bleeding.
7. Dip a cotton bud in rose water, and dab it on the inside of the nostrils to stop bleeding.
8. Mix nutmeg powder with milk and apply on the forehead and nose to stop a 'runny' rose.
9. Mix crushed garlic with honey and lemon juice in water, and drink this to stop watery discharge.

Obesity
1. Take two glasses of water just before meals.
2. Drink a glass of water mixed with lemon juice and honey every day.
3. Mix three teaspoons of lemon juice, a teaspoon of honey and a quarter teaspoon of pepper powder in a cup of water, and drink this for three months.
4. Eat 10 curry leaves every morning.
5. Eat a tomato before breakfast.
6. Eat a small piece of ginger with honey every morining.

Oedema
1. For swollen ankles, massage with a solution of castor oil and lemon juice.
2. Drink a cup of warm water mixed with lemon juice and honey.

Peptic Ulcer
Swallow a teaspoon of fenugreek seeds on an empty stomach in the morning. Then drink a cup of chilled milk in which two crushed cardamoms have been added.

Piles
1. Apply Vaseline with boric powder on the anus to stop itching.
2. Mix bittergourd juice with buttermilk and sugar candy, and drink it first thing in the morning.
3. Drink onion juice mixed with ghee and sugar.
4. Eat an onion that is chopped and added to curds.
5. Boil a mashed banana in a cup of milk. Take it twice a day.

6. Mix curry leaves juice with honey and drink it twice a day.
7. Consume fresh radish every morning.
8. Add a quarter teaspoon of carom seeds and rock salt to buttermilk, and drink it twice a day.
9. For bleeding piles, drink milk mixed with half a teaspoon each of poppy seeds, neem leaves juice and pomegranate flower powder.
10. Soak three figs overnight in water. Drink it first thing in the morning.
11. Mix equal quantities of mint juice, lemon juice and honey, and take it thrice a day.
12. Take an infusion of coriander seeds with milk and honey.
13. Take black cuminseeds with water.
14. Add a teaspoon of mango peel paste to a cup of buttermilk, and drink this thrice a day.

Prickly Heat

1. Apply the water that is used to wash raw rice, on the body.
2. Apply a thick solution of coconut oil mixed with cumin seed powder on the body. Bathe after 20 minutes.
3. Splash rose water over the body.
4. Mix rose water with sandal paste, and apply on affected parts.

Prostate Problems

1. Follow basically a healthy diet, and increase zinc-containing foods such as seafod (especially oysters), pumpkin seeds, eggs and brewer's yeast. Lean meat also contains zinc.
2. Reduce intake of fried foods and most vegetable oils.

3. Eat organically-grown vegetables if possible, as pesticides can reduce zinc absorption.
4. Eat oily fish such as salmon, mackerel, sardine and herring at least thrice a week.
5. Drastically reduce, or better still, eliminate alcohol, especially beer,
6. Cut down your sugar and caffeine (coffee, tea, cocacola) consumption.
7. Drink at least one and a half litres of clean water per day.
8. Eating half a cup of pumpkin seeds a day helps. Pumpkin seeds are beneficial for the treatment of mild to moderately enlarged prostate glands.

Ringworm
1. Apply unripe papaya slices on the ringworm patches.
2. Apply the milk oozing out of a plucked mango from the tree on the affected parts.
3. Apply the juice of basil leaves on the patch.
4. Apply a paste made from mustard seeds and water.
5. Apply a paste of nutmeg mixed with one's own saliva.

Scabies
1. Apply a solution of caraway oil, alcohol and castor oil.
2. A paste of tamarind leaves can be applied over scabies with beneficial results.
3. Apply the fresh juice from turmeric rhizomes on the scabies.
4. Apply a solution of basil oil, lemon juice and onion juice.
5. Mix turmeric powder and pepper powder with gingelly oil, and apply on the scabies.

6. Apply a solution of sandal paste and buttermilk on the scabies.
7. Combine neem leaves paste with turmeric powder and apply on the affected part.

Sexual Debility
1. Drink an infusion of ground fenugreek seeds mixed in one cup of water.
2. Eat a teaspoon of onion seeds (*kalaunji*) thrice a day.
3. Take at night a semi-boiled egg with half a teaspoon of ginger juice and honey.
4. Take a quarter teaspoon of nutmeg with honey and a half-boiled egg an hour before going to bed.
5. Drink a cup of milk mixed with half a teaspoon of pepper powder and eight crushed almonds.
6. Take milk with saffron twice daily.
7. Eat gingelly with jaggery.
8. Take three teaspoons of dry pomegranate seeds with milk.
9. Take roasted cuminseeds with honey.

Snake and Scorpion Bites
1. Apply a paste of cumin powder and onion juice on the scorpion-stung area.
2. Apply a paste of as asafoetida and lemon juice over the scorpion sting.
3. Place a crushed garlic flake on the sting.
4. Chew basil leaves, and drink the water in which is combined paste of basil leaves, and pepper powder, if bitten by a snake.

Spleen Problems

For an enlarged spleen, burn the bark of a peepal tree and mix the ash with a little potassium nitrate. Take a spoon of this every day.

Sprains

1. Mix garlic juice with coconut oil, and apply on the sprain.
2. Foment the area with roasted hot salt tied in a cloth.
3. Put ice cubes in a polythene bag and apply on the sprain.
4. Mix almond oil and garlic oil in equal proportions, and massage over the sprain.
5. Mix butter with the paste of lemon leaves and apply on the affected area.
6. If you have sprained your ankle, soak it in water to which a few drops of lavender oil have been added.

Stomachache

1. Mix the juices of mint, ginger and lemon with black salt, and take it on an empty stomach.
2. Mix a paste of fenugreek seeds with buttermilk.
3. Take a pinch of asafoetida with a teaspoon of ghee.
4. Grind guava leaves with cuminseeds, and take a spoon of this when you have stomachache.
5. Swallow a teaspoon of carom seeds and a pinch of salt with warm water.
6. Mix a teaspoon each of mint juice and lemon juice with a quarter teaspoon of ginger juice and a pinch of black salt. Drink this.
7. Take a teaspoon of basil juice mixed with lemon juice.
8. Make a paste of five tender leaves of peepal tree with an equal quantity of jaggery. Take this paste twice a day.

9. Boil a piece of ginger in a cup of water for two minutes. Mix it with fruit juice and drink it.
10. Take a teaspoon of ghee with garlic juice.

Thirst
1. Tender coconut water mixed with sandal paste is an excellent drink to quench one's thirst.
2. Mix a teaspoon of sandal powder in a cup of milk, and drink this.
3. Eat tender mango with salt.

Throat Problems
1. Eat the tender leaves of the mango tree to clear throat ailments.
2. For a sore throat, gargle with a solution of salt water and soda bicarb.
3. Swirl a solution of two teaspoons of glycerine and a teaspoon of borax powder for a while in your mouth before swallowing it.
4. Drink a hot infusion of juice of two lemons, a piece of crushed ginger and a teaspoon of sugar in a quarter cup of water for a sore throat.
5. Take an infusion of hot mint water mixed with honey.
6. Drink a hot cup of milk to which is added half a teaspoon each of turmeric powder and pepper powder.
7. Chew basil leaves first thing in the morning.
8. Gargle with a warm solution of honey and neem juice.
9. Drink tea boiled with ginger and a few basil leaves thrice a day.
10. Heat six cups of water with two tablespoons of fenugreek for 20 minutes on a low flame. Strain and gargle often with this.

11. Gargle with hot ginger water.

Tuberculosis
1. Sip a little bit of the mixture of a teaspoon each of butter, sugar, candy and honey.
2. A teaspoon of ginger juice mixed with a cup of fenugreek infusion is an excellent medicine in the treatment of tuberculosis.

Typhoid
1. Eat a mashed banana with a tablespoon of honey.
2. Drink a cup of buttermilk mixed with two teaspoons of coriander leaves juice.

Ulcers and Boils
1. Apply a grated potato on boils.
2. Apply a paste of cloves on boils.
3. Mix bittergourd juice with sugar and apply on the ulcer.
4. A hot poultice of turmeric powder lessens the pain of an abscess.
5. Mix wheat flour, honey and turmeric powder and heat slightly. Tie in a muslin bag and tie the hot poultice on the boil. This brings out the pus and heals the skin.
6. Apply ground neem paste on the affected parts.
7. Boil fenugreek leaves and eat with honey.
8. Mash a garlic and apply on the boil.
9. Mix black cumin powder in water and apply the paste on the boil.
10. Heat pepper powder in ghee till charred. Apply as ointment on the boils.
11. Apply a paste of ginger and turmeric on the boils.

Urinary Problems

1. Barley water removes the burning sensation in the urine, and helps the free flow of urine.
2. Eat a lot of ashgourd to prevent urinary problems.
3. Eat plenty of cucumber.
4. Drink gooseberry sherbet to stop blood being discharged with urine.
5. Drink tender coconut water to remove the burning sensation while passing urine.
6. Eat a mashed banana mixed with a tablespoon of gooseberry juice.
7. Take an infusion of tender papaya leaves.
8. Take basil juice mixed with honey and lemon juice.
9. Take buttermilk with fenugreek seeds.
10. Drink water with mint juice for painful urination.
11. Take milk with two teaspoons of pomegranate seeds.
12. For scanty urination drink cardamom tea.

Vomiting

1. Drink the juice of basil leaves with cardamom powder.
2. Soak coriander seeds in water, and take it in sips.
3. Drink water with cardamom powder added to it.
4. Chew a small quantity of cuminseed.
5. Drink the whey water after removing the paneer from curdled milk.
6. Lick slowly the fried clove powder-honey paste.
7. Suck a piece of ice slowly.
8. Suck sliced ginger.

Warts
1. Mix betel leaf juice with lime, and apply on wart.
2. Apply onion juice.
3. Apply nail varnish on it once every day until it dries up and disappears.
4. Apply crushed garlic on the wart, and after an hour, wash with cold water. Repeat two-three times a day.
5. Apply pineapple slices on warts.

Whitlows
1. Mix pepper powder with milk, and apply.
2. Mix lemon juice and turmeric powder. Apply on whitlow and bandage it.
3. Make a hole in a lemon and fill it with ginger and salt paste. Insert the affected finger into it and allow the pus to come out.

Chapter Two
Skin Care

Abrasives
1. Combine together lemon juice, sugar and glycerine to make an effective facial abrasive.
2. Massage in a teaspoon of sugar along with Pears soap. This mild abrasive removes dead cells from the surface of the skin, leaving the skin clean and glowing.

Acne
1. Each time you wash your face, use sugar to scrub it, at least once a day, for two weeks, to rid yourself of acne.
2. Soak cotton wool in mint juice, and apply every day.
3. Apply crushed marigold leaves on acne.
4. Boil and mash plums to get about eight teaspoons of pulp. Add a teaspoon of almond oil, and apply on the face.
5. Make a paste of turmeric powder, and apply evenly on the acne.
6. Mix together neem leaves paste, a quarter teaspoon of turmeric powder, sandalwood paste and gram flour. Apply on the acne and let it dry well before rinsing.
7. Powder half a cup of whole green gram. Mix it with two tablespoons wheat bran. Regular application of this will clear the skin of acne.

Blackheads

1. Apply a paste made of Fuller's earth (*multani mitti*) and rose water on the face. When dry, rub with a coarse cloth to dislodge impurities.
2. Soak cotton wool in pure lemon juice, and apply on problem areas.
3. Cleanse your face with unboiled milk. Gently rub a coarse cloth dipped in milk to remove the blackheads.
4. Rub oatmeal paste on face. Leave it to dry for 15 minutes before washing off with cold water.
5. Soak a face napkin in a solution of one and a half cups of hot water and one teaspoon of boric powder. Press this napkin on the face. Repeat. Extract blackheads with a blackhead remover and sterilised cotton.
6. After a facial steam, apply warm honey on affected areas. Rinse off after 15 minutes.

Bleaches/Bleaching

1. For bleaching your face, mix together two tablespoons of milk and juice of one lemon. Apply on face and neck, and massage for a few minutes. Rinse off.
2. Mix equal parts of lemon juice and cucumber juice. Apply on face and after five minutes rinse off. This acts both as an astringent as well as a bleach.
3. Grind oatmeal to a fine paste. Add a spoon of lemon juice. Apply on darkened areas, and leave to dry. Wash off, and lightly rub on some moisturiser.
4. Apply a paste made of almond paste, cream and lemon juice every day to bleach hands.
5. Mix together one teaspoon of honey, one and a half teaspoons of cream, and one teaspoon of lemon juice. Apply on face and wash off with lukewarm water.

Blemishes

1. Mix together half teaspoon of olive oil and quarter teaspoon of lemon juice. Apply on the blemishes, and after 15 minutes wash off.
2. Grind a sprig of mint leaves, and add a teaspoon of rose water to it. Apply it at night and wash it off the next morning. Or else, apply it during daytime, and wash off after two hours.
3. Add neem leaves to a bucket of water. Boil and reduce to three-fourths of the original quantity. Strain and cool. Apply on the affected smallpox marks or other blemishes thrice daily.
4. Add a little carrot and orange juice to a cup of milk. Rub this on the smallpox-scarred face, and in course of time the marks will gradually disappear.

Complexions

1. Soak four almonds at night. Peel off the skin and grind the nuts into a paste. Add one and a half teaspoons of gram flour, one teaspoon of fresh raw milk, and four drops of lime juice. Apply even on the face. After 15 minutes gently massage the face till the dried mixture it comes off. Rinse with warm water, then splash cold water on the face. This will help to lighten a dark-complexioned skin.
2. Massage the face with fresh coconut water every morning for about 10 minutes for a fairer complexion.
3. Mix a teaspoon of gram flour with a pinch of turmeric powder, a few drops of lime juice, quarter teaspoon of olive oil and milk. Apply on face and leave for half an hour. Wash off with water. Constant practice of this is belived to improve the complexion.

4. Cut slices of a raw potato and keep them in cold water for a few minutes. Then rub these slices over your face to make it fairer.
5. Reverse an empty milk sachet. Gently rub the creamy milk residue on your face, neck and forearms. After 10 minutes wash off with warm water. This works as an excellent skin softener and whitener.
6. An effective treatment to clear complexion is a mixture of gram flour and cucumber juice rubbed over face, neck and arms.
7. Mix sandalwood paste and turmeric powder with a few drops of lemon juice. Apply a thick coat on the face, and wash off after half an hour. This will enhance your complexion.
8. A paste made of sandalwood and rose water may be applied every day.
9. Cucumber juice is considered to be an excellent whitener.
10. Gently massage coconut water all over the face and neck to lighten your skin.
11. Make a paste of almonds and rose water and apply on face. Wash off after 10 minutes.
12. Coconut milk and cucumber juice in equal quantities make your skin fairer.
13. Deseed and mash grapes. Apply liberally over face and skin. Wash off after 15 minutes.
14. Combine together equal quantities of salt and baby oil. Rub gently on face to slough away rough, dull skin.
15. Boil neem leaves in water, and allow to steep before washing your face with it for a better complexion.
16. Apply undiluted orange juice with a cotton pad all over the face and neck. Wash off after 15 minutes.

17. Add nutmeg powder to icy cold water, and splash your face with it to get your complexion glowing.
18. Rub honey on your face, wash it off after 10 minutes. This brings lack the glow to your face.

Deep Cleansing

Pour boiling water in a bowl, and add the herb of your choice. Cover head and cool with a towel and steam your face. It is specially suited for an oily skin.

Freckles

1. To get rid of freckles, add a teaspoon of lemon juice to some buttermilk. Dip cotton wool in this, and pat it on the face. Leave until dry, then wash it off.
2. Combine a teaspoon each of buttermilk and lemon juice, and a tablespoon of radish juice. Apply on face, and let it dry before rinsing off.
3. Remove the skin of an apple. Mash it well and apply on the freckles every day.
4. Make a smooth paste of oatmeal powder and buttermilk. Apply on the freckles, and leave for 20 minutes. Wash off with cold water.
5. Make an almond paste with three ground almonds, an egg white and a teaspoon of lemon juice. Apply on freckles, and when dry, wash with tepid water followed by splashing cold water.

Pimples

1. Smear a little camphor lotion on the pimples daily. Wash off with lukewarm water and a medicated soap.
2. Apply mint juice on the pimples. Allow to dry before washing off.
3. Use sandalwood paste with undiluted cucumber juice on pimples.

4. Mix together one tablespoon of gram flour, half a teaspoon of turmeric powder, one teaspoon of neem juice, and enough milk to make a smooth consistency. Leave on for 20 minutes before washing off.
5. Dab a little starch paste on the pimple at bed time, and wash it off in the morning.
6. Apply a mixture of sandalwood oil and mustard oil on pimples.
7. Make a paste of Fuller's earth and rose water. Apply on the face and leave for 15-20 minutes. Rinse off with lukewarm water.
8. Mix sandalwood paste and cucumber juice. This application will discourage pimples.
9. Apply the paste made from fenugreek on pimples at night. Wash with warm water the following morning.
10. Mix sandalwood powder and half a teaspoon of turmeric in a little raw milk. Apply on the face for half an hour daily before taking a bath.
11. Rub the skin with orange peel, or half a potato.
12. For corn-like pimples on dry skin, massage face with gingelly or coconut oil.
13. Daily application of sandalwood paste on the face prevents pimples.
14. Add the juice of coriander leaves to turmeric powder and apply on pimples.
15. Mix lemon juice, rose water and glycerine in equal quantities. Apply daily before retiring to bed.
16. Applying toothpaste to pimples twice daily clears your skin.
17. Soak crushed neem leaves in hot water, then boil. Apply on the pimples while still warm.

18. Mix an equal quantity of eau-de-cologne and boiled and cooled lemon juice. Apply over pimples, and wash off after 20 minutes.
19. Apply a curd-gram flour mixture. After 15 minutes, wash off.
20. Wash your face with raw milk before going to bed to prevent pimples.
21. Use jasmine petals-curd mask. Grind the petals and mix with curd. Apply, and leave to dry for 20 minutes. Wash off.
22. Mix cinnamon powder with lime juice to make a fine paste. Apply on pimples.
23. Wash your face with coconut water daily to prevent pimples.
24. Grind a piece of the bark of a neem tree. Mix it with turmeric powder and apply on pimples.

Skin

1. To keep skin soft, massage with a solution of gingelly oil, mustard oil and olive oil. After an hour, you may bathe.
2. To prevent dryness in winter, use gram flour instead of soap.
3. Massage the skin with the fruit pulps of papaya and over-ripe bananas. Leave on for 10 minutes. This removes dead cells, and produces enzymes to make the skin glow.
4. Egg pack is ideal for all types of skin. The white is ideal for oily skins, yellows for dry, and the entire egg for a normal skin. Add two drops of lemon juice for oily, and a few drops of olive oil for dry skin.
5. The juice of a tender potato may be applied to keep the skin free of eruptions.

6. A mixture of lemon juice and water, applied on the skin with cotton pads, yields good results.
7. To make the skin healthy and glowing, apply a mixture of egg yolk and almond oil.
8. Throw in starch in your bath water, for that extra soft and smooth feel.

Skin, dry

1. Dissolve a little yeast in cabbage juice. Add a teaspoon of honey, mix well and apply it thickly over your face. Leave for 15 minutes, then rinse.
2. Make a paste with two teaspoons of Fuller's earth, one teaspoon each of honey and rose water. Add a few drops of glycerine. Apply and leave for 15 minutes. Wash, and gently massage two drops of vitamin E oil.
3. Apply olive or almond oil on your face and massage with fingertips. Do this before going to bed.
4. Make a cleansing mask using half a teaspoon each of brewer's yeast and vinegar, two tablespoons of sour cream, 2 yolks, one tablespoon of honey and milk. Spread a thin film of olive oil on face. Then apply this mask. After 20 minutes rinse off with milk and water.
5. Yoghurt-honey combination helps dry skin.
6. Make an egg face pack with a yolk, a teaspoon of honey, a tablespoon of milk powder. This is beneficial to dry skin types.
7. Apply a face pack made of one tablespoon olive oil, half a lemon and a yolk.
8. An ideal facial pack for dry skin is a mixture of almond and olive oil.

Skin, oily

1. Rub a lemon rind over your face to lessen grease and to bring a glow to your complexion.
2. Add a spoon of rose water and a few drops of lemon juice to a few spoons of cucumber juice. Apply on the face for improving an oily and dull complexion.
3. Apply the white of an egg on the face. After 10 minutes, wash your-face with warm water.
4. A tablespoon of honey mixed with an egg white is a nourishing and drying mask for an oily skin.
5. Mix together equal quantities of rose water, lettuce juice and lemon juice. Apply an hour before bath.
6. Make a cleansing mask for an oily skin by combining a quarter cup of oatmeal powder, half a cup of yoghurt, and two teaspoons of lemon juice.
7. Make a tomato mask consisting of a tomato, the rind of half a lemon, and a dash of lemon juice.
8. Make a yeast mask, by mixing one teaspoon of brewer's yeast and two tablespoons of yoghurt.
9. Make an oatmeal mask with a tablespoon of oatmeal powder, half a tablespoon of lemon juice, and three teaspoons of milk.
10. Combine a teaspoon of cucumber juice, half a teaspoon of lemon juice, and three drops of rose water. This remedies a greasy skin.
11. Make a gram flour mask with one tablespoon gram flour and two tablespoons of cucumber juice.

Sunburn

1. Lime juice, added to a little milk, is a good remedy against sunburn.

2. For sunburns, mix two teaspoons of tomato juice with four tablespoons of buttermilk. Spread on the affected area, and leave for half an hour. Wash off.
3. Pamper your skin with an application of vitamin D ointment.
4. Use olive oil or peanut oil for relief from sunburn.
5. Grate and squeeze a cucumber. Spread the seeds and juice over the sunburnt area.
6. Make an anti-sunburn lotion. Whisk an egg white, transfer contents into a pan, and simmer on a low fire till it thickens. Add the juice of one lemon. Apply on the sunburn and do not wash off.
7. Boil lettuce leaves in a cup of boiling water to get a strong infusion. Apply on the sunburn.
8. Use whey on the sunburnt skin.
9. Yoghurt with honey helps to cool and promote healing in sunburnt skins.

Suntan

1. Add a little rose water to lemon juice. Apply on the face overnight. Wash in the morning.
2. Soak a cotton pad in buttermilk and apply. This is a good remedy to remove suntan.
3. Combine equal quantities of olive oil and vinegar. Apply and keep it for at least two hours before bath.

Wrinkles

1. Spread a mixture of honey and carrot juice on the face. Leave it on for 20 minutes. Add a pinch of soda bicarb in a little warm water. Soak a cotton pad in it and remove the mask.
2. A piece of papaya pulp mixed with a dash of cream helps in combating wrinkles.

3. Gently massage the face with glycerine-honey mixture.
4. A banana pack consisting of a ripe banana and rose water prevents wrinkles.
5. A mixture of honey and a few drops of orange juice can work wonders for a mature skin.
6. Dip a cotton pad in unbeaten egg white, and smooth it across wrinkles. Leave it on for an hour. Remove it with a cotton dipped in ice-cold water.
7. To remove only wrinkles, apply the paste made of two teaspoons of green gram flour, a few drops of coconut oil and a pinch of turmeric. Apply, and wash with cold water after 20 minutes.
8. Spread a mixture of glycerine and unbeaten egg white on wrinkled areas. After 15 minutes rinse with tepid water.
9. Massage a mixture of glycerine and honey.
10. Make an anti-wrinkle mask with one and a half tablespoons of honey, half a teaspoon of carrot juice, and a pinch of soda bicarb.
11. Make a cream mask by combining the white of an egg and a tablespoon of cream.
12. Prepare a cornflour mask using equal quantities of cornflour and honey.
13. Mask apple, and use as a facial mask to postpone wrinkles.
14. For a banana mask, mix a tablespoon of rose water with a ripe masked banana.
15. An anti wrinkle mask consisting of a teaspoon of cucumber juice, an egg white, a tablespoon of mint juice, half a teaspoon of honey, and a teaspoon of curd is ideal for removing wrinkles.
16. Mix an egg and a teaspoon of olive briskly. Apply on face and allow to dry. Soak a cotton pad in hot water to which soda bicarb has been added. Gently clean the skin surface.

Chapter Three
Care of Face and Neck

Face
1. Tomatoes cut in half and rubbed over the face are useful in toning up and whitening the skin, and refining pores.
2. To give a velvety smoothness to your skin, just throw in a little starch to your bath water.
3. For a good complexion, wash your face in the morning with rain water stored in glass jars.
4. Clean the face with cotton pad soaked in raw milk. Rub the face gently with it from the chin upwards to the hairline.
5. For a supple skin, put a spoonful of ground nutmeg in a bowl of water, and splash this over the face.
6. Apply a solution of lemon juice and basil leaf juice on the face. Allow it to dry, and wash off.
7. Grated raw potato applied to the face keeps the face cool and smooth.
8. Mix a little lemon juice with barley powder and milk to form a thick paste. Apply this on the face, and let it stand for 15 minutes to get a lustrous and glowing skin.
9. Massage your face with a mixture of equal parts of baby oil and table salt to remove dead surface skin and to soften the skin.

10. The paste of fenugreek seeds blended with boiled milk is an effective cosmetic for a smooth skin.
11. A teaspoon of gram flour mixed with cream, sandal paste, and turmeric powder to form a paste and applied on the face half an hour before bath is an excellent beauty aid to keep the face fresh and soft.
12. Drink the juice of basil leaves mixed with a little honey twice a day for a glowing face.
13. For men, who have rough and hard skin due to frequent shaving, apply a 20 per cent solution of hydrogen peroxide in water with a cotton pad.
14. Use a mixture of lemon juice and glycerine (in equal quantities) as an excellent substitute for cold cream.
15. Rub the leaves of ridgegourd on the face a couple of times daily to remove dark patches from the face.
16. If you have hollow cheeks, try massaging gently in slow, circular movements from mouth and chin upwards towards the ear with warm almond oil. This will, to a certain extent, bring fullness to your cheeks, as it is a rich and nourishing oil.
17. For a lustrous and glowing skin, apply the paste made with dry basil leaves powder and a little water. Leave it on for one to two hours before washing your face.
18. A little rouge blended into the chin and eyelids will help to give length to a round face.
19. Grind dry lime rinds with bengal gram dal (*chana dal*). Store in the fridge. When required, mix with curd, and leave on face for 10 minutes. Wash off with warm water.
20. Grind some rose petal with sandalwood. Apply on face. After 10 minutes wash off. Your skin will be bright and soft.
21. Rubbing ice on the face is healthy for the skin.

22. Beat a yolk with one tablespoon of olive oil. Smooth the mixture over your face, and leave for 20 minutes. Wash with warm water, patdry, and dab on eau-de-cologme.
23. Beat two tablespoons of lemon juice, one yolk and one tabespoon of honey till it thickens. Apply and leave until it dries. Rinse well.
24. Apply a tablespoon of raw papaya paste on the face, and leave for 15 minutes. Rinse off to get a clear skin.
25. Make a paste of two almonds, two tablespoons of milk, one tablespoon of carrot juice, and one tablespoon of orange juice. Apply a thick coat on the face, and leave for half an hour. Wash off. It will leave your face tingling and glowing.
26. Yoghurt and mashed cucumber have a toning and freshening effect.
27. Egg white with yoghurt softens the skin.

Facial Masks
1. Make a mask that is ideal for a sensitive skin, as well as useful to rid eruptions like acne. Mix together almond, sandalwood, egg white, honey, and yoghurt into a paste and apply on the face.
2. Milk cream mask is another great mask. With a few drops of lemon juice in raw milk, the mask brightens up dull, sallow and dry complexion. It is best to apply it half an hour before bath.
3. Beat the white of an egg until stiff. Add five tablespoons of yoghurt. Apply it on the face. Wipe clean with a soft towel dipped in hot water, followed by dipping it in cold water. For oily skin, add a teaspoon of lemon juice. For a dry skin add a teaspoon of honey.

4. To make turmeric cleansing mask, combine one and a half teaspoon of turmeric powder and one and a half tablespoon of lemon juice.
5. For an oatmeal mask, mix one tablespoon of oatmeal with enough milk to make a paste. Beat a yolk and blend it into a paste. You can substitute glycerine for yolk.
6. For a cleansing mask, mix together equal quantities of oatmeal and cucumber juice.
7. To prepare Fuller's earth mask, mix two tablespoons of crushed Fuller's earth (*multani mitti*) and three tablespoons of milk.
8. Extract the juice of a potato, and add Fuller's, earth to make a thick paste.
9. Cucumber juice mixed with Fuller's earth helps to cleanse dirt that is embedded deep in the skin.
10. Boiled and mashed turnips mixed with a little yoghurt is a good cleansing mask.
11. Mashed strawberries have excellent cleansing properties.
12. Regular application of ripe, mashed papaya on the face leaves the skin clean, smooth and shining.
13. Carrot mask containing the juice from a half carrot, and a quarter teaspoon honey is excellent for a sensitive skin, as carrot has plenty of vitamin A.
14. Avocado mask made of the pulp of a quarter avocado, a beaten yolk and half a teaspoon of honey is a perfect one for dry skin.
15. Potato mask comprising one tablespoon raw grated potato and half a tablespoon of curd is an ideal mask for a dry skin.
16. To make a simple oatmeal mask, soak one and a half tablespoons of oatmeal in a little milk and water for 15 minutes.

17. Cucumber mask made of half cup mashed cucumber, the white of an egg, and two teaspoons skimmed milk powder is ideal for a sluggish and tired face.
18. Beat an egg and one teaspoon honey for a dry skin, and lemon juice instead of honey for an oily skin.
19. Prepare honey mask by combining one tablespoon each of Fuller's earth, honey and rose water, and 10 drops of orange juice.
20. Use parsley mask consisting of one bunch of parsley leaves (pureed) and one tablespoon of honey for a combination skin.
21. Honey and egg mask, having an egg, a teaspoon each of sesame oil and honey gives tone and elasticity to the skin.
22. Make starch mask with one tablespoon starch and water. Massage your face with a little olive oil. Then apply the mask, and leave for 20 minutes. Rinse off thoroughly with warm water.
23. Barley face mask has equal quantities of barley powder, milk and lemon juice.
24. Honey face mask can be made with half a teaspoon each of honey and barley into which is added a frothy egg white.
25. Make an egg mousse facial mask with an egg white, one teaspoon cream and a quarter teaspoon of castor sugar, all beaten well.
26. To prepare an all-purpose mask, mix together a teaspoon each of curd, lemon juice, carrot juice and gelatine (dissolved in water), two teaspoons brewer's yeast, and half a teaspoon each of barley powder and olive oil. The fruit and vegetable juices supply minerals and vitamins, barley gives protein, yeast stimulates blood flow, and curd cleanses the skin.

27. Make an almond mask with four almonds soaked in water and grounded, and mixed with two tablespoons of milk, one tablespoon of orange juice, and the contents of one vitamin A capsule.
28. Grated raw papaya makes an excellent mask for a blemished skin.

Facial Packs

1. The cream of milk makes a good facial pack.
2. Fuller's earth pack is good for an oily, large-pored skin. Mix together one and a half tablespoon each of Fuller's earth and lemon juice, and half a teaspoon of honey.
3. Make banana honey pack with half a banana and half a tablespoon of honey.
4. Make a winter pack of one tablespoon of wheat germ mixed with olive oil to make a paste.

Nose

1. Dab on some cucumber juice before applying foundation or powder. This will give a smooth effect on the nose.
2. Tweeze the inner corners of the eyebrows to counteract the upturned shape of the nose, or a very short nose.
3. For a long nose, the hair of your eyebrows should be tweezed to form a line at a decided angle to the line of the nose.
4. To offset a broad or puffy nose, apply a darker shade of powder on the sides of the nose, and a light shade in a line down the centre. Blend well with your usual foundation.

Pores

1. Ice wrapped in cotton wool, and rubbed gently on the face closes open pores.

2. Add a grain of camphor to beaten egg white. Mix well and spread this mixture over the face, then rinse well.
3. The fresh juice of cucumber and honey, are equally beneficial.
4. Massage tomato pulp on the face to close open pores. Tomatoes have astringent and anti-tan enzymes.
5. Soak a cotton pad in buttermilk. Pat over face and allow to dry. Rinse off.
6. Apricot with tomato pulp is an excellent pore shrinker.
7. Equal quantities of tomato juice and buttermilk rubbed on the face shrinks the large pores.
8. Lettuce leaves juice and a few drops of lemon juice make an excellent pore tightener.
9. Soak five almonds for an hour. Grind and mix with a teaspoon of lemon juice. Apply on the face. After 15 minutes rinse off with tepid water.
10. Clean your face with warm water. Apply two tablespoons of milk of magnesia. Rinse off after 20 minutes, with tepid water, then cold water.
11. Rub half a lemon over the entire face, and allow it to dry. Wash off.

Neck

1. Mix the juice of a lemon with a little oatmeal or gram flour. Apply on the neck and leave for 15 minutes. Wash it off. This takes care of wrinkles, and whitens the skin.
2. Mix together rose water, glycerine and egg white. Apply over neck. Allow to dry before rinsing off. This is excellent for lined and wrinkled necks.
3. To bleach and smoothen dry skin on the neck, rub the pulp of an avocado with lemon juice.
4. Rub pure cucumber juice to bleach the neck.

Chapter four
Mouth, Teeth and Chin Care

Bad Breath/Mouth Washes
1. Freshly plucked basil (*tulsi*) leaves are natural mouth fresheners if chewed and kept in the mouth for some time.
2. Blow air through the nozzle of an empty toothpaste tube. Fill it half with water and shake well. Makes an excellent mouthwash.
3. To stop bad breath, gargle with warm water to which is added the juice of half a lemon.
4. Chew a couple of cloves to remove bad breath.
5. Gargle with mint juice.
6. Chew on an orange peel for half an hour.
7. A little tamarind combined with salt and rubbed on the tongue cleans it and reduces bad breath.
8. Mix equal quantities of water and vinegar, and use as a rinse.
9. Gargle with rose water.

Double Chin
1. Chewing gum reduces facial wrinkles and even eliminates a double chin.
2. Apply olive oil under chin and along throat. Start with strokes from the base of the throat to the jawline. Tap

with light pressure on the double chin, and then stroke. Keep alternating.

Gum
1. To strengthen gums, chew roasted sesame seeds with jaggery. This also helps to keep the teeth shining and healthy.
2. To strengthen gums, cleanse your mouth with salt water after brushing your teeth.

Lips/Lipsticks
1. Thin lips or broad lips can be corrected by outlining them with a lip pencil, a little outside or inside the natural lip line. Apply lip gloss on the upper lip for giving a full appearance to your lips.
2. Outline crooked lips either below or above the natural shape depending on the fault.
3. If you have full and thick lips, line your lips inside the natural shape with a lighter shade of lipstick, and fill in the outline with a shade lighter.
4. Lipstick with a matt finish helps to give the illusion of smaller lips. To get a matt finish, place a thin tissue over the lips after applying lipstick, then remove.
5. If your lip line is droopy, outline it upwards with the lip pencil in a shade slightly darker than your lip colour. Use lip gloss to touch up the centre.
6. Rub almond oil regularly on your lips to keep them from chapping.
7. In winter, apply a little cream or butter on the lips before going to bed, to prevent your lips from chapping.
8. Apply honey on lips to keep them moist. It is good for chapped lips.
9. While applying lipstick, use a brush to spread it evenly on the lips.

10. Before applying lipstick, put a thin coating of powder on the lips so that the lipstick stays on for a longer time.
11. To mend a broken lipstick, join both the broken ends with a toothpick, and store in the fridge for a day.
12. Bright lipstick makes the mouth appear larger.
13. Lip pencils will be easier to sharpen if popped into the fridge for about 15 minutes.
14. Take a few old lipsticks, and scoop out their contents. Put them into a spoon. Hold the spoon over a low flame. When it melts, put back in a container, and leave in the fridge. The result is a fantastic, new shade.
15. A tip for only men! Eucalyptus oil removes lipstick marks from clothes!

Teeth

1. A little baking soda or coarse salt put on your toothbrush or paste will make your teeth pearly white.
2. Using your fingers, rub a mixture of soda bicarb and lemon juice on your teeth for a sparkle in them.
3. Eat an apple after meals to give a fresh sparkle to your teeth.
4. To prevent tooth decay, brush your teeth with a mixture of alum powder and salt.
5. Brush your teeth, using the powder of dried lemon rinds. This cleans and whitens your teeth, and is also a good mouthwash.
6. Baking soda can be used instead of toothpaste when you have run out of the latter.
7. Mix soda bicarb and hydrogen peroxide equally. Rub on teeth for shining teeth and removal of the yellowish coating on teeth.

8. If your teeth have turned yellow, rub corking soda on the teeth as often as possible.
9. Use the inner part of an orange peel to rub teeth for a lovely, white shine.
10. Use a slice of a strawberry or apple to rub your teeth and bring out their whiteness.
11. Chew crunchy carrots and celery leaves.
12. An excellent whitener is a combination of orange peel powder and powdered bay leaves.
13. Rub teeth with dried neem leaves powder to clean your teeth.
14. Equal quantities of soda bicarb and salt lend teeth a bright sparkle.

Chapter five
Care of Eyes

Crow's Feet
1. Olive oil or petroleum jelly applied gently on the crow's feet daily will help to replace lost moisture, minimise lines and fight possible new ones.
2. Potato compressed over closed eyes fights the formation of the wrinkles on the outer corner of eyes.
3. To get rid of the fine lines around eyes, brush cold egg white on the lined area, and wash off with ice-cold rose water when dry. The lines will gradually fade away.

Dark Circles
1. Cover your eyes with cotton soaked in lukewarm milk for 15 minutes every day to remove the dark circles around your eyes.
2. Peel and deseed a cucumber and grate it. Remove the juice and tie the pulp in a muslin cloth. Gently pat the dark circles around the eyes with it, for 10 minutes. Wash off your face after this. Use the cucumber juice as an astringent for the face.
3. To reduce dark circles under the eye, mix one tablespoon of milk with one tablespoon of fresh potato juice. Chill it in the fridge. Apply it around your eyes, and allow to stand for 10 minutes before washing off.

4. Cut out two slices of apple, and keep them on your closed eyelids for 10 minutes.
5. Dip cotton pads into freshly extracted mint juice. Flatten them and place them on closed eyelids for 10-15 minutes. Wash off the areas.
6. Soak cotton pads into cucumber lemon juice solution, and keep the flattened pads on the eyelids for 10-15minutes.
7. Apply half a teaspoon of almond oil with a quarter teaspoon of lemon juice.

Eyes
1. Apply a little Vaseline to your eyelids to get a luminous look. This will prevent the eyelids from drying, and will help the lashes to grow.
2. In order to have bright, sparkling eyes, just splash cold water on them every morning.
3. If your eyes are sleepy or dull-looking, place thin slices of cucumber on the eyelids for 10 minutes.
4. To rejuvenate dull and sleepy eyes, add a pinch of salt in a cup of ice-cold water. Soak two cotton pads in it and squeeze them. Keep them on the eyelids for 10 minutes.
5. Remove eye make-up with a piece of cucumber. It is safe, and helps to keep the eyes cool and fresh.
6. A solution of ice-cold water and a tablespoon of rose water can be used to wash eyes.
7. Wash eyes with a mild solution of salt water. Pat dry with a very soft towel.

Eyes, deep set
1. If your eyes are too close together or deep set, remove enough hair from the inner corners of the eyebrows to create at least an inch of space between the eyebrows.

2. For deep set eyes, use lots of mascara, and to make the eyes look larger, apply a blue eye-liner along the inside of the lower lid.

Puffy Eyes

1. Reduce puffiness under eyes by applying pads dipped in a solution of one litre water and one tablespoon salt.
2. You can camouflage the puffiness by a clever application of make-up. Use a darker than skin tone foundation on the puffy area, and then apply your usual foundation blending it well.
3. To reduce puffiness under eyes, dip two metal spoons into a glass of iced water. Lay a damp cotton material over each eye, then place a spoon over this, and leave for 10-15 minutes.
4. Dip two cotton pads in ice-cold milk. Place them over the eyelids and relax for 10 minutes.
5. After splashing the eyes with ice-cold water, place a potato slice on each eyelid for 10 minutes.

Eyes tired

1. Revive tired eyes by soaking two cotton pads in chilled water to which a few drops of eau-de-cologne have been added. Place them on your eyelids for 10 minutes, and relax.
2. Mix together equal parts of cool water and lemon juice. Soak cotton pads in it and place on eyelids for 10 minutes.
3. A drop of pure castor oil in each eye soothes tired and srained eyes.
4. To relax tired eyes, place a slice of cucumber on each eyelid for 10 minutes.
5. Keep a wet teabag on each eyelid for 10 minutes to soothe tired eyes.

6. Grate a potato. Place the shreds in two muslin bags and place them on the eyelids for 10-15 minutes.
7. A little chilled water with a pinch of salt can be used to soak two cotton pads, which can be placed on the eyelids.
8. Pads soaked in chilled rose water and placed on eyelids relive tired eyes.

Eyebrows

1. In order to darken your eyebrows, smooth a little castor oil in them.
2. For scanty eyebrows, add a few drops of glycerine to a little castor oil, and apply it on the eyebrows. Leave it on overnight. It may take about six weeks to show any improvement.
3. Leave your eyebrow pencil in the fridge overnight, and it will sharpen easily.
4. Before plucking eyebrows, lay a hot flannel over the area for several minutes to open the pores, and make plucking the hairs easier.
5. Petroleum jelly brushed daily over the eyebrows with a toothbrush will help maintain their shape.

Eyelashes

1. Apply castor oil to your eyelashes before retiring every night to make them grow longer, darker and thicker.
2. To make your sparse eyelashes look thicker, powder the lashes before applying mascara. Let the mascara dry. Then repeat.
3. For the good growth of your eyelashes, apply almond or olive oil on them regularly at night.

Mascara

1. If your mascara tends to look clotted, brush your lashes with an old toothbrush after applying mascara. This separates the lashes, clears out the clots, and gives the lashes a natural look.
2. Fill used mascara bottles with castor oil. Apply it every night on your eyelashes.
3. To remove mascara place a roll of cotton wool under top eyelashes, and then wipe them with another piece of damp cotton wool.
4. Two or three thin coats of mascara on the eyelashes look more natural than one thick coat.
5. Apply baby powder or talcum over each back lid, and then apply the eye shadow. The powder will give the eye shadow a firm non-greasy base on which to stick.

Chapter six
Hair Care

Baldness
1. Hair washed with the paste of fenugreek seeds prevents baldness.
2. Neem oil applied regularly on the bald patch on the scalp will promote hair growth.
3. Make a paste of three baby onions, three peppercorns and half a teaspoon of salt. Apply on the affected area.

Combs/Hairbrushes
1. Used toothbrushes can be used with soap and water to clean combs.
2. To remove the dust from a comb quickly, sprinkle a little soap powder and water on it. Hold the comb and scrub it with an old toothbrush.
3. Combs can be cleaned by dipping them for a while in a solution of washing soda and warm water.
4. If you are attending a party, and have not had time to wash your hair, dip your comb in a glass of beer and comb well.
5. Never use a brush on a wet hair as it will only tear it. Instead, use a wide-toothed comb.

Dandruff

1. Massage your scalp with warm coconut or castor oil twice a week. Leave it overnight and shampoo the following morning.
2. Wash hair with the paste of fenugreek seeds.
3. To remove dandruff, soak equal quantities of fenugreek and cumin seeds overnight. Grind to a paste with milk and massage on the scalp well, then wash well.
4. If you cook rice directly and drain the water, use that water for treating dandruff. Wash off with green gram powder, and then clear water.
5. Apply lemon juice with the rind well on the scalp. After five minutes wash off with shampoo and water.
6. Mix one tablespoon pure vinegar in half a bucket of water. Shampoo and wash well. Rinse finally with the vinegar solution.
7. Massage sour curds on the scalp. Leave it for half an hour, then shampoo it.
8. Mix a tablespoon of lemon juice with two tablespoons of coconut oil. Massage it into the scalp. Leave it for more than an hour, then wash with warm water.
9. Powder 15 peppercorns and mix it with cow's milk into a paste. Apply on the scalp twice weekly, keeping it on for 10 minutes each time before washing your hair.
10. Take equal quantities of jaggery and tamarind. Grind into a paste. Apply on scalp and wash it off after 10 minutes.
11. Soak four tablespoons of gram flour in a little vinegar for 15 minutes. Apply on scalp and leave for about half an hour, then rinse.
12. Mix together two yolks with two teaspoons of water. Wet hair, apply this mixture on the scalp, and rub well. Wash with hot water.

13. Massage a handful of soda bicarb into the scalp and rinse thoroughly.
14. A herbal rinse is a safe method of removing dandruff. Make a basic infusion by adding four tablespoons of fresh parsley in nearly a litre of boiling water. Simmer for 15 minutes. Leave for three hours and then strain.
15. Make a basic infusion of celery leaves. When cool, add lemon juice/vinegar, and rinse your hair with it.
16. Make a basic infusion of mint leaves. When cool, use it as final rinse.
17. Boil one tablespoon of tea leaves in nearly a litre of water for three minutes. Cool and use it for a final rinse.
18. Combine two tablespoons of freshly squeezed lemon juice with 800 ml of ice-cold water. Rinse your hair finally with it.
19. Collect and strain whey. Use it as a rinse for dandruff.
20. Fill a muslin bag with four tablespoons of powdered oatmeal. Soak the bag in a litre of water for four hours. Squeeze the bag to extract the milky white liquid in the water, and use as a protein rinse.
21. Mix four tablespoons of whey with four tablespoons of camphor water. Apply and wash off after three hours.
22. Application of brandy on the scalp is said to clear dandruff.
23. Extract thick coconut milk with hot water, and add lemon juice. Apply on the scalp and allow to remain there for half an hour. Rinse off with tepid water.

Hair, dry

Massage olive oil, once a month, well into the hair. Cover your head with a hot towel, and leave for several hours. Then shampoo as normal.

Hair Drying

Never blow dry hair when they are wet, for intense heat only promotes broken ends. Instead, towel dry as much as possible.

Hair, greying

1. Regular massage of gooseberries (amla grounded into a paste) on the scalp does wonders in reversing the process of greying.
2. To prevent early greying of hair, add a tablespoon of salt to a cup of strong tea. When cold, strain, and apply it to the roots. Leave for an hour, then wash it off. Don't shampoo.
3. To check greying of hair, mix lemon juice in castor oil. Beat till frothy. Add mehendi powder. Apply on scalp, and wash off after an hour.
4. Soak 12 rithas and 4 shikakai pods in water overnight. In the morning, boil and strain. Use as a normal shampoo. Soak 12 amlas in a cup overnight. Strain and use as a conditioner. Leave it on for 10 minutes, then rinse hair. This stops premature greying of hair.
5. Heat coconut oil. Add three flakes of garlic and three peppercorns. Cool and apply on scalp.
6. Mix starch from cooked rice with a little gramflour, and apply to the scalp. Wash after a few minutes.
7. Massage your scalp with a few tablespoons of mayonnaise, and rinse with water. This keeps your hair lustrous and prevents greying.
8. Mix two yolks, two tablespoons of olive oil, and two tablespoons of rum. Apply to the hair and scalp, and leave for an hour. Rinse off.
9. Heat 250 gms castor oil and 50 gms olive oil. When warm, add 50 gms sandalwood powder, 50 gms amla powder and 50 gms coffee powder. Keep stirring till the oil separates

from the residue. Massage this oil into the scalp, and leave it overnight.

10. Premature greying of hair can be postponed by using a strong decoction of black tea and a tablespoon of salt. Strain and apply to roots for 45 minutes. Wash with water. Don't shampoo.
11. Make a paste with ground curry leaves and sour buttermilk. Use this once a week.

Hair, brittle

For brittle hair, combine one cup curd, of lemon two teaspoons of henna, a teaspoon of lemon juice, and two teaspoons of oil. Massage into the scalp and leave for half an hour. Wash off with regular shampoo.

Hair, Oily

Do not brush greasy hair. Instead comb it. Brushing encourages the glands to secrete more oil.

Hair, thin

1. For thin hair, perming makes your hair look bulky.
2. Garlic, crushed and massaged into the scalp, increases blood circulation, and prevents thinning of hair.

Hair oils

1. Clip off the tips of green grass, and soak them in coconut oil. Warm the oil in the sun. Massaging the oil into the scalp improves hair condition.
2. Soak hibiscus flowers in coconut oil, and keep them in the sun. Use the oil regularly to massage the scalp.
3. Heat a cup of coconut oil with eight crushed peppercorns and 15 basil leaves. Use this every day.

4. For an itchy scalp, heat coconut oil with a few crushed peppercorns, a good pinch of cuminseeds, and a red chilli till it smokes. When slightly cool, apply on the scalp and rinse after 10 minutes.

Hairspray

For a natural finish to your hairstyle, put hairspray on to the brush, and then run the brush over your hair.

Hair Loss

1. Rub oil into the scalp. Wring out a towel in hot water and wrap it on the head. Keep it on for 15 minutes. Shampoo and dry well.
2. To treat hair loss apply a little lemon juice with used tea leaves or coconut milk.
3. For hair loss, massage with coconut oil in which fenugreek seeds have been soaked.
4. Beat two eggs, and add two tablespoons of water to it. Rinse hair and pour the egg mixture over the hair. Massage the scalp well, and leave for 10 minutes. Then wash it.
5. Mix together coconut milk (got from half a coconut) and lemon juice. Massage into scalp, leave for half an hour, and rinse with warm water.
6. Washing hair with a weak solution of salt cleans the scalp, cures dandruff, and prevents hair loss.
7. Shampoo hair regularly with shikakai, amla and reetha nuts.
8. Massage whipped egg white all over the scalp. Allow to dry, then wash off.
9. Make a thick paste of fenugreek seeds, and wash hair with this.

Hair Tonic / Conditioner / Shampoo

1. The use of hot and cold water alternating quickly acts as a great tonic for both hair and scalp.
2. A few drops of glycerine will bring clarity to turbid shampoo.
3. Add water to leftover tea leaves and boil. Cool and strain. Use the water as a last rinse to make hair shiny and silky.
4. A few drops of lemon juice added to the bath water will give a shine to your hair.
5. After shampooing, give your hair a final rinse with water in which walnut shells have been boiled.
6. Soak shikakai seeds, reetha and dried amla overnight in the proportion of 2:2:1. In the morning, boil for 15 minutes. Remove the seeds, and blend the pulp in a mixer. Refrigerate and use when needed.
7. Apply sour buttermilk to your hair, and wash off after 15 minutes with warm water.
8. Grind together basil leaves, hibiscus leaves and flowers to a fine paste. Use this as a shampoo and conditioner.
9. Break eggs and dry in the sun. Powder and keep them in the fridge. When required, mix with soapnut powder (reetha) and wash hair. This makes an excellent conditioner.
10. Use vinegar rinse to soften hair. It acts as a good conditioner.
11. As you apply shampoo to your hair, add the white of an egg. Lather well, and rinse thoroughly until there is no slipperiness whatsoever between your fingers and hair.
12. Grind equal quantities of whole green gram and fenugreek seeds with hibiscus leaves. Make a paste with gram flour and the water left over after cooking rice. Wash hair with this effective home-made shampoo.
13. A good substitute for shampoo, if you run out of it at the last minute, is men's shaving cream.

14. A handful of hibiscus leaves grounded to a paste with a teaspoon of shikakai is a wonderful shampoo and conditioner.
15. Boil three handfuls of celery leaves. Remove the leaves, and add the juice of a lemon to it. Makes an excellent conditioner.
16. A mixture of gram flour and curd makes a good shampoo and conditioner for long and lustrous hair.
17. Mix gooseberry paste with sour buttermilk. This is an affective shampoo-cum-conditioner.
18. In between washing your hair, freshen your hair up by rubbing cologne-soaked balls of cotton into the scalp.
19. When washing children's hair, prevent shampoo running into their eyes by smearing a band of petroleum jelly over their forehead.
20. Put some milk in a spray bottle. Spray on the hair when damp, and leave for 20 minutes. Then rinse off with shampoo. This straightens the hair and gives it a shine.
21. Mix together two cups of henna, one cup of water, one teaspoon of lemon juice, and one tablespoon of coffee powder. Apply and leave for half an hour for conditioning, and three hours for dyeing the hair. Rinse with water, then shampoo it off.
22. Beat a yolk well in a quarter litre of water. Add a drop of vanilla essence to counteract the smell of egg.
23. Make an egg shampoo using one egg and the juice of one lemon.
24. Mix together three tablespoons of henna, two tablespoons of strong coffee, one egg, one teaspoon ground cloves, two teaspoons parsley leaves paste and half a teaspoon of castor oil. Use this as a conditioner.

Hair, superfluous
1. Application of turmeric paste daily during a bath improves the complexion, and arrests the growth of superfluous hair.
2. For treatment of unwanted hair on the body use a pumice stone with soap and water (not on face).
3. Apply a spoon of moistened gram flour on the face. Rub with a dry cloth the area where there is unwanted facial hair. Wash the face as usual.
4. Apply the ashes of incense sticks mixed with sour curds. Application of this arrests hair growth.
5. Heat three tablespoons of turmeric powder in three and a half tablespoons of coconut oil. Apply for arresting growth of unwanted hair.

Lice
1. To get rid of lice, apply a paste of dried and powdered apple seeds and water to your hair. Rinse after half an hour.
2. Grind half a kilogramme of custard apple leaves with water to a fine paste. Apply and rub into scalp. Dry for 45 minutes and then wash off.
3. To get rid of lice, apply the juice of basil leaves to the hair, leave overnight, and then wash off.
4. Keep basil leaves or camphor below the pillow to get rid of lice from the hair.

Hair, split ends
Regularly massage warm castor oil into your scalp and hair to prevent split ends.

Chapter seven
Care of Arms and Hands

Elbows
1. Rub elbows with warm olive oil to smoothen them.
2. Discolouration of the skin of elbows can be treated with the help of a pumice stone.
3. To bleach the elbows, cut a lemon in half, and place your elbows into each half for 15 minutes.
4. To remove the dryness from around the elbows, give it a regular treatment with a moisturising cream.
5. To clean your elbows and soften the skin, rub them regularly with a mixture of broken wheat (*dalia*), milk cream and lime juice.
6. To lighten the colour of the elbows, apply a mixture of milk cream, turmeric powder and ground basil leaves, and leave for a few hours before washing them off.
7. Put a drop of oil on a lemon rind, and rub it on the dark elbows.
8. A few drops of baby oil rubbed on the elbows smoothens them.
9. Add enough lemon juice to a little powdered oatmeal to form a paste. Apply on hands, and rinse after it dries.

Fingers

Stains on the fingers, if rubbed with vinegar before the hands are washed, will soon disappear.

Hands

1. Rub corn-meal in between soapy palms to give your hands a friction bath.
2. Clean stained hands with a teaspoon of salt mixed with olive oil. Massage this on hands, and rinse well.
3. A paste made of ground almonds, a few drops of lemon juice and glycerine, and milk cream is very effective for bleaching hands.
4. Mix a teaspoon of lemon juice with a few drops of cold tea. Rub on the palms to ward off perspiration in the hands.
5. To smoothen hands, rub the paste of granulated sugar-lemon juice between the palms. Rinse off after five minutes.
6. After emptying the milk vessel or the milk sachet, rub your hands inside it.
7. Lemon juice mixed with rose water and glycerine makes an effective hand lotion.
8. Rub a slice of tomato over your arms twice or thrice a day. Wash after each application. On the following day, massage the juice well into your skin. When dry, wash off with borax-mixed water. Mix glycerine and rose water and pat on arms. Blot off excess with a tissue.
9. To soften hands, apply a paste of a ripe tomato pulp, lemon juice and glycerine, and massage well. Leave for half an hour, and wash.
10. Application of glycerine and lime juice on hands at bed time ensures softness.

11. Remove ink stains from hands by rubbing lightly with a cloth dipped in ammonia. Rinse immediately.
12. For any stains on hand, rub with lemon or raw potato.
13. To brighten dark hands, apply a mixture of rose water, glycerine and lemon juice.
14. For soft and smooth hands, rub a little olive oil on your hands before retiring to bed.
15. For dry hands, rub salt mixed in oil on hands, and wash with soap after 15 minutes.
16. For chapped hands, apply vinegar, and pat dry.
17. Apply glycerine to hands during winters to keep them smooth.
18. Apply baby oil before retiring at night.
19. Smoothen your hands by applying a coat of yoghurt. When dry, wash off.
20. Use petroleum jelly for hand massage.
21. Mix together two teaspoons of olive oil and one and a half teaspoon of lemon juice. Massage well into hands.
22. Wet your hands. Gently rub bran over them. Rinse off for that extra smooth soft hands.
23. Mix together equal quantities of orange juice and honey. Leave on hands for 20 minutes, and rinse off with tepid water.
24. Add a few drops of glycerine to three tablespoons of rose water. Its application leaves your hands soft and silky.
25. Apply a paste of almond on dry hands. After 15 minutes wash off with warm water.
26. Make a protein paste with one teaspoon each of olive oil, lemon juice and glycerine, two tablespoons of oatmeal and one tablespoon of milk. Excellent for making hands soft.

27. Combine lemon juice with tomato pulp and a few drops of glycerine. Use it to soften hands.

Mehendi

1. To remove pale and old mehendi marks from your hands, rub a raw bottlegourd (*ghiya, lauki*) on your hands.
2. Disposable syringes are an excellent substitute for mehendi cones.

Nails/Nail Polish

1. Brittle nails can be strengthened by dipping the fingers in olive oil at bed time.
2. Cut up an old sponge into pieces. Use them as toe separators while painting your nails.
3. Nail polish, if stored in the fridge, will last for a year.
4. If your nails are brittle, place your fingers in softened soap every now and then.
5. To keep the nails shining and glowing, apply sandalwood oil daily.
6. Soak cotton pads in raw milk, and rub on nails to shine them.
7. For strong nails, soak your finger in a solution made of half a cup of hot water, two teaspoons of mustard oil, and one teaspoon of salt.
8. To prevent the cap of a nail polish bottle from getting stuck to the bottle, add a little oil inside the cap before screwing it on to the bottle.
9. To melt hardened nail polish, add a few drops of eucalyptus oil, and keep it for a day.
10. To open jammed nail polish caps, hold the bottle in front of a running hair dryer for a few seconds.

11. Dip your fingers in warm olive oil for about 10 minutes, then massage it. This strengthens the nails.
12. To dry nail polish on your fingers if you are in a hurry, dip your hands in cold water for a few seconds.
13. A few drops of lemon juice added to water will give an extra shine to the nail polish.
14. Before pushing cuticles back, warm up some hand lotion, and soak the nails in it for five minutes. This helps in pushing the cuticles back.
15. After removing nail polish from the fridge, stand it upside down for half an hour.
16. Before involving yourself in a messy job, press nail into petroleum jelly to prevent dirt getting lodged under the nails.
17. Nicotine-stained fingers can be cleaned by rubbing with smoker's toothpaste.
18. To strengthen weak nails, use extra hardening varnish on them.
19. Dip your wrists and fingers into a bowl of milk for 10 minutes. Pat dry. This can be done once a week.
20. Use an abrasive cleanser of one tablespoon granulated sugar in seven drops of vegetable oil. Massage it over and under the nails to slough off dirt embedded in them.
21. Make a nail cream by combining a teaspoon each of avocado pulp, egg yolk, honey, and a pinch of salt. Massage gently on to nails, and rinse off after half an hour. This cream softens the cuticles.
22. Trim your nails with a nail clipper, cutting them straight across.

Chapter Eight
Care of Knees and Feet

Knees
1. To a tablespoon of milk of magnesia, add a few drops of lemon juice. Leave on knees till dry. Wash, dry and apply a little moisturiser.
2. Rub your knees with a paste made of wheat bran or husk, milk cream and lime juice to smoothen them.

Feet
1. Soak feet in warm soapy water. Wash, clean and dry. Rub a little olive oil to prevent cracking of the skin on the feet.
2. Freshen tired feet by plunging them into alternate bowls of warm and cold water, ending with cold. A handful of salt thrown in the last bowl of cold water will do wonders to your tired feet.
3. If milk curdles, strain it. Rub the thick paste on your feet. Wait till it dries well. Wash off with tepid water, and dry. The grime comes off, leaving your feet soft and smooth.
4. Rub your ankle with a lemon rind to give an extra softness and shine to the skin.
5. Treat dry skin on feet with a pumice stone. Rub glycerine on them at night.

6. Walking barefoot at home relaxes tired feet.
7. Soak your feet in a bowl of warm water in which Epsom salt is added to relieve tireness.
8. Dust talcum powder over bare feet during a hot, sticky weather, and they are less likely to cling to sandals.
9. Before shaving legs, smooth baby oil over them for silky, smooth legs.
10. To reduce swelling in your feet, cut a potato in half. Rub over feet in a circular motion. Allow to dry, and leave overnight. Wash them in the morning.
11. Before retiring for the night apply two tablespoons of lemon juice mixed with one and a half tablespoons of glycerine.
12. Soak your feet for 15 minutes in hot water to which is added a tablespoon of mustard. Wash off with cold water.

Heels
1. Use a pumice stone to rub off dead skin, and smoothen heels.
2. Rub lemon halves to bleach heels.
3. Rub a mixture of Vaseline and lemon juice on heels to soften them.

Toes
Rub lemon halves on toes, toenails and between toes to keep your feet bleached and sparkling.

Chapter Nine
Beauty Aids

Astringents
1. Rose water makes a good astringent when applied with the juice of a lemon.
2. Yoghurt combined with tomato pulp serves as a good astringent.
3. Combine equal parts of vinegar and water to get an effective astringent.
4. Tomato juice rubbed over the face is a good and economical astringent.
5. Satuarate cotton wool in pure lemon juice, and apply as astringent.
6. Mash a small peach and add four drops each of lemon juice and tomato juice to make an astringent lotion.

Baths
1. Precious drops of olive or almond oil added to your bath water enhances a creamy, shiny and smooth skin.
2. To prepare a rich oil bath, blend together a quarter cup of olive oil, one tablespoon shampoo, one cup vegetable oil and one tablespoon lemon juice. Use one or two tablespoons for your bath.

3. Add 30 gms of Epsom salt to your bath, and soak in it for 20 minutes. This bath helps to neutralise waste materials present in the body tissue. It also helps to open clogged pores.
4. Add five tablespoons of milk powder to bath water, to nourish and soften the skin.
5. In a muslin bag fill three tablespoons each of skimmed milk powder, oatmeal powder and laundry starch. Immerse this bag in a bucket of water till the water turns milky. Bathe with this water for a clear and glowing skin.
6. Throw a couple of lemon peels into the bath for that tangy, refreshing feeling.
7. A tablespoon of honey adds more moisture to your bath, and leaves your skin dewy and fresh.
8. Tie oatmeal in a muslin bag, and place it in a bucket of water for five minutes. While bathing, massage your skin gently with it. You will feel a sense of being well scrubbed.
9. Add a handful of salt to your tub, and soak in it for 10 minutes. You will feel rejuvenated.
10. Tie herbs in a piece of cloth and let it soak in your bucket of hot water till you get the beautiful fragrance. Bathe with this water for a relaxed feeling.

Creams/Lotions/Tonics
1. Mix two teaspoons each of gram flour and curd with two pinches of turmeric powder. Apply on the body, rub well and bathe in warm water.
2. Mix together four teaspoons of barley powder, three teaspoons of turmeric and coconut or mustard or gingelly oil to make a paste. This can be used on the body, and for the face dilute it with raw milk.

3. Gram flour mixed with turmeric powder and olive oil makes an excellent cream.
4. To two teaspoons of boiled and mashed masoor dal, add a teaspoon of rose water. Add fresh cream. This cream brings a natural glow to the skin.
5. To prepare orange skin cream for natural glow and softness of skin, dry orange peels and powder. Before bathing, make a paste of two spoons of it with raw milk, and massage on body before bathing in warm water.
6. Mix mustard seed paste in raw milk. Apply on body and rub in well. As it starts drying and falling off from the body, bathe in warm water. This cream helps to remove wrinkles and fissures on your skin.
7. Mix together two teaspoons each of almond paste and chironji paste with a little milk. Applying this cream on the body makes the skin soft, glowing and beautiful.
8. Lemon cream makes your skin glow and also improves your complexion. For this mix together the juice of lemon, one and a half teaspoons of gram flour, two pinches of turmeric powder, a little coconut oil and cream.
9. Mix a teaspoon of lemon juice and half a teaspoon of honey with a few drops of milk. This lotion has a mild bleaching effect on a greasy skin.
10. To one tablespoon of cucumber juice, add a few drops of lemon juice, and a pinch of turmeric powder. This lotion makes on excellent whitener for all types of skins.
11. Water melon lotion is ideal for clearing the skin of all blemishes. Grate and squeeze juice out of a small piece of water melon. Apply on face and leave on for 15 minutes, then wash off with cold water.
12. Keep the shell of an egg soaked in boiling water for half an hour. It serves as a good tonic for a dull skin when washed with water.

13. Any sun cream left over can be used as a body lotion if you don't want to keep it till the next year. Once opened, sun cream deteriorates and loses its protective qualilities, yet retains its moisturing ingredients.
14. For extra protection during summer, choose a foundation cream containing a sun cream.
15. Make a sunscreen lotion at home. Extract the juice of one medium-sized cucumber, add half tablespoon each of glycerine, water and milk, and refrigerate.
16. To make a natural astringent lotion, mix together one teaspoon of peach juice, half a teaspoon of carrot juice and a quarter teaspoon of lemon juice. Apply on face and neck and leave for 15 minutes. This will tighten the skin without robbing it of its natural oils.
17. An effective substitute for cold cream is equal parts of lemon juice and glycerine mixed together.
18. Soak two tablespoons of oatmeal overnight. In the morning, mix it with one tablespoon lemon juice, half a teaspoon each of diluted ammonia, olive oil, rose water, glycerine and four tablespoons of warm water. An excellent hand lotion.
19. Another effective lotion is a mixture of three tablespoons rose water, two tablespoons lemon juice and one tablespoon glycerine.
20. Mix together two and a half teaspoons each of honey, glycerine and barley powder, one egg white, and four tablespoons of rose water, into a thick paste. It is good for the hands.
21. Use generously on hands the paste made of one and a half teaspoon each of almond oil and petroleum jelly, one teaspoon lemon pulp, two and a half teaspoons each of glycerine and lemon juice.

22. Prepare a rich conditioning cream by combining 125 gms lard, one tablespoon each of honey, ground almonds and rose water, six drops of almond essence, and two yolks.

Dyes

1. If you want to dye your hair red, add a spoon of glycerine to a cup of water in which the outer skin of an onion has been boiled. Use this on your hair, and after half an hour, rinse.
2. To remove dye stains on skin, mix together an equal quantity of utensil cleaning powder and Dettol. Rub the stained area with this, and wash with water.
3. To get instant colour in henna, break open an iron capsule, and add its contents to the henna mixture. It will lend a rich, deep brown tint.

Foundation

1. A few drops of moisturiser added to foundation will make it easier to apply.
2. Apply foundation with a slightly damp sponge for a better finish.

Moisturiser

1. To remove dead skin from the face, apply a mixture of glycerine, lime juice and sugar, and rub gently. Then apply a little cream or glycerine.
2. Add a glass of milk to your bath water. The milk protein helps in softening dry and wrinkled skin.
3. Massage your face with a little honey every day to keep the skin smooth. Honey is a good and natural moisturiser.
4. For a dry skin, use a few drops of wheat germ oil as a moisturiser.
5. Use almond oil moisturiser on a sensitive skin.

6. Add a splash of bath oil to the bath water. This prevents the skin from drying.
7. Lighten base make-up with a touch of moisturiser.

Perfume

1. To allow the perfume to set before stepping outdoors, apply perfume at least 20 minutes earlier.
2. To give a lovely smell to your clothes, add a little perfume into your steam iron.
3. Rub perfume on the palm of your hand, then press the palm in the nape, on your wrists and elbows, and on the hairline of your elbow.
4. Smear a drop of Vaseline on the areas where you would like to dab on your perfume. The scent will linger for long hours.
5. Leave unscrewed used perfume bottles among your lingerie for that lovely smell.
6. Soak a small pad of cotton with perfume, and pin it up inside your clothes or dress for the scent to waft around you.
7. A little perfume in the hair goes a long way.
8. Soak leftover pieces of bath soap in warm water. Wash your handkerchiefs in the soapy water for a mild perfume.
9. If you have not had the time to wash your hair before attending a party, freshen it up by dabbing cologne on to the hair roots.

Scrubs

1. Mix together equal quantities of oatmeal powder, wheat germ powder, skimmed milk powder and one teaspoon sandalwood powder. Tie in a muslin bag. Dip in warm water and gently rub on the face and neck for at least 15 minutes in circular movements. Wash off with tepid water.

2. Make an orange peel scrub by mixing four tablespoons powder, and two tablespoons wheat germ powder.
3. Combine four tablespoons of green gram powder, and two tablespoons each of gram flour and sandalwood powder for an excellent scrub.
4. Make a complexion scrub with a tablespoon each of ground almonds and orange peel powder, and one-teaspoon ground oatmeal.
5. Make an oatmeal scrub with two tablespoons each of oatmeal powder and grated Pears soap, and a tablespoon each of almond oil and vegetable oil.
6. Prepare green gram scrub with ten tablespoons of green gram powder, five tablespoons of oil and two tablespoons of orange peel powder. When using it, add rose water.
7. Rub the peel of oranges or lemons all over the body, and bathe, to get that soft, extra-smooth skin.